The Three-Edged Sword

Being Ill in America

Maureen Audrey Potts
The University of Texas at El Paso
El Paso, Texas

UNIVERSITY PRESS OF AMERICA

Lanham • New York • London

4720 Boston Way
Lanham, Maryland 20706

3 Henrietta Street
London WC2E 8LU England

Printed in the United States of America
British Cataloging in Publication Information Available

Library of Congress Cataloging-in-Publication Data

Potts, Maureen A. (Maureen Audrey), 1941–
The three-edged sword : being ill in America /
Maureen Audrey Potts.
p. cm.
Includes bibliographical references and index.
1. Potts, Maureen A. (Maureen Audrey), 1941– —Health.
2. Systemic lupus erythematosus—Patients—United States—
Biography. I. Title.
RC924.5.L85P68 1992 362.1'9677—dc20 92–9197 CIP

ISBN 0–8191–8669–4 (cloth : alk. paper)

To the ill of America

ACKNOWLEDGEMENTS

I wish to thank my friend and colleague, G. Douglas Meyers, who first suggested I write this book and who encouraged me throughout its long evolution. My friend Donna Reardon read the manuscript in its early stages and has been a constant source of support. Other friends and colleagues who sustained me while this project was evolving include Mary Trejo, Dennie Watts, Theresa Melendez-Hayes, Lois Marchino, Mimi Gladstein, Leslie Ullman, Gail Mortimer, Roberta Walker who taught me about hyphenating compound nouns and adjectives, and Evelyn Posey who taught me how to use a laser printer. I am particularly grateful to Dale Walker of Texas Western Press who shared with me his vast knowledge of the publishing business and to Nancy Hamilton who gave me invaluable editorial advice and the title. In addition, I would like to thank Robert Bledsoe, chair of the English Department at The University of Texas at El Paso, for providing me with technical support. The late Arturo Islas was also encouraging when I most needed it and I deeply regret he did not live long enough to see it in print.

I also owe an immeasurable debt of gratitude to Jary Jones, who sustained me during the bad times, likewise to Charlie and Sue Zaltz, and above all to Richard Patterson, friend and companion, who generously wrote the Foreword.

Finally, I would like to thank my family, especially my mother and father, for accepting my illness and for encouraging me to help others by writing about it.

CONTENTS

FOREWORD

A revolution of sorts appears to have gripped the American medical scene, born, as are all revolutions, of dissatisfaction, discontent, and anger. The battles are being fought in hospitals and physicians' consulting rooms everywhere. We American consumers have grown unhappy with many aspects of the medical care we receive. We are unhappy with the cost of health care. We are unhappy with the remote and impersonal attitudes of health-care professionals. We are unhappy to learn that our medical deities do not always have answers. And so we are speaking up. The impact, the success, of this revolution is still in doubt, in part because most of the alternatives which are being developed do not address a central issue--the patient's own responsibility.

Dr. Maureen Potts' journey with lupus as recounted in *The Three-Edged Sword* is in part a modern horror story as she recounts uncaring treatment, an absence of answers and the difficulty practitioners typically have in acknowledging their lack of answers. Her book, however, is not a tale of bitterness. We see with each encounter her growing awareness that she needed to place herself at the center of her diagnosis and treatment. In other words, she realized how much she (and we) displaced responsibility to physicians, and she took steps to reclaim that responsibility. That awareness is one which needs to be central in the aforementioned revolution. In this era of alternative medicines, we see patients everywhere turning away from physicians and seeking out gurus, curanderas, faith healers, and other non-traditional sources of help in their search for answers. In this trend, the basic challenge of responsibility is in danger of being over-looked. It is this responsibility for our own health care which Dr. Potts challenges us all to face.

I remember once when I had gone to my physician to have some blood drawn to see why my fingers went numb in the cold. He called me with the results several days later and vaguely referred to the blood tests being normal. When I mentioned this to Dr. Potts, she asked me, "Do you know what tests he ran? Did you request a copy of the results?" When I had to admit no to both questions, I realized how I had avoided the responsibility of understanding the workings (and breakdowns) of my own body and had passed that responsibility over to my doctor, when, with the help of a good medical dictionary, I could probably have figured it out for myself.

Dr. Potts' insights and observations of the medical community may not be well-received by health-care professionals. This would be unfortunate since she does not encourage us to turn to alternative medicine for answers. She simply asks us to take charge of our own medical care and asks health-care professionals to encourage, even to insist on, our acceptance of this responsibility.

Beyond this theme of responsibility, and perhaps far more important, Dr. Potts' journey is testimony to the importance of addressing the psychological and spiritual as part of one's attitude towards health. As she examines her dreams, struggles with old hurts within the context of religion, faces depression, struggles to remain active as a teacher and writer, we see the delicate and complex interplay of body, mind, and spirit--a complexity Dr. Potts encourages us to embrace.

Finally, Dr. Potts' book is a rare, first-hand account of the evolution of a genuine Wounded Healer. She faces her woundedness, learns and grows from it, then draws on that body of information to reach out to others. She does so with compassion and humility.

The Three-Edged Sword is a work for those battling illness. It is a work for health-care professionals and for professionals-in-training. It is a work for psychotherapists no matter what their specialty. Most importantly, it is a work for those in need of a reminder of the magnificence of the human spirit in facing suffering. And in the midst of the debates which this book may generate about the pros and cons of medicine, we must not forget that it is, first and foremost, an intensely personal story of one woman's efforts to heal while at the same time keeping the wolves of loneliness and despair at bay.

Richard B. Patterson
Clinical Psychologist and author of *In Search of the Wounded Healer*

INTRODUCTION

In November of 1985, I was diagnosed as having systemic lupus erythematosus (SLE, more commonly referred to as lupus), a chronic and currently incurable autoimmune disease that can affect virtually any part of the body. For some unknown reason, people with autoimmune diseases produce abnormal antibodies that attack their own body tissue, mistakenly identifying it as an invading enemy. In some of these diseases, the renegade antibodies attack specific tissue as in the case of multiple sclerosis (the myelin sheath around the nerves), rheumatoid arthritis (the collagen tissue in the joints), and polymyositis (the muscles). In systemic lupus, however, the confused immune system can and does attack any of the soft tissue in the body, including the heart, lungs, liver, kidneys, and the connective tissue--skin, muscles, ligaments, tendons, and the lining around the major organs.

The disease strikes mainly young women in their childbearing years, although anyone can fall victim, and is characterized by a vast array of symptoms. The most common complaints are weakness and debilitating fatigue, nausea, diminished appetite and weight loss, chronic low-grade fever, pain, general muscle and joint aching, and frequent infections. In addition, lupus patients also manifest a striking sensitivity to the sun. They experience a severe rash, nausea, and weakness on exposure to the sun, and in the particularly sensitive patient, to any form of ultraviolet rays. The most obvious trademark of lupus, while not occurring in all cases, is the butterfly rash over the nose and face of the sufferer.

These symptoms do not always occur with all patients and come and go with maddening unpredictability. When the disease is slumbering, the symptoms subside and are almost unnoticeable, lulling the sufferer into a false sense of security. However, any kind of medical event such as an allergy attack, the 'flu, surgery, anything that causes the immune system to become activated, can and often does lead to a "flare." Stress, overwork and fatigue will have the same result, and what is even more frustrating, a flare will sometimes strike for no apparent reason. What makes the disease so difficult to diagnose is that during times of remission, all laboratory findings are usually negative, and it is not until the patient goes into a flare that the clinical evidence re-emerges. If the patient presents herself to her physician during a time when the disease is merely smoldering, her lab tests will probably come back negative, leading the doctor to mistakenly assume a psychosomatic illness. Because the disease can manifest itself in so many ways and can affect so many different organs, it has often been dubbed "The Great Imitator," confusing even the most diligent physician who has not been trained to recognize lupus.

THE THREE-EDGED SWORD

Until the recent flurry of research into the immune system, lupus was considered inevitably fatal, usually within five years after diagnosis. Indeed, if the present-day patient runs to outdated books, she will find lupus defined as a fatal disease of young women. The outlook for most lupus patients is now a normal life span with occasional flares, but with long periods of months, even years, in remission. One cause for the statistical turnaround is the better diagnostic procedures which are now identifying the milder cases. In addition, the new anti-inflammatory drugs, especially corticosteroids, have done a marvelous job of controlling the disease and keeping the symptoms to a minimum.

Only recently have researchers begun to speculate on the causes of lupus and other autoimmune diseases. They are now beginning to think it has something to do with genetics and with DNA structures, that people who develop faulty immune systems have some kind of specific genetic marker or defect that makes them susceptible to immune disasters. And others are speculating on the notion of an as yet undetected virus that makes the immune system get its signals crossed, or perhaps even environmental factors such as pollution and the depletion of the ozone layer. We now know a great deal about the AIDS virus and while not an autoimmune disease, much of the research into that illness is beginning to provide answers for these other diseases. But we are still on the frontiers of medical science in our understanding of the human immune system.

In the following pages, I have recounted my sixteen-month, twenty-doctor search before I was given the diagnosis of lupus, and my struggles since as I have been forced to live with chronic illness. My story, however, is not about lupus, although I obviously have much to say on the subject. It is about coping with disease in the context of our current cultural attitudes about illness, and it is about coping with the complex economic, social and rhetorical demands of our health-care system. The three-edged sword, the central metaphor of this work, describes the set of miseries ill people in twentieth-century America must endure, and which I hope my story illustrates. On the one side, every patient must endure the physical and psychological discomforts of disease itself, discomforts that do not respect national boundaries and do not discriminate between the rich or poor, black or white, male or female. These include pain, weakness, nausea, general debilitation, and the side effects of drug therapy which often include hair loss, nausea, bloating, constipation, diarrhea and dizziness. And intimately tied up with the physical are the psychological blows of depression, ego-deflating dependency, the loss of self-esteem that comes with the destruction of physical appearance, anger, fear, anxiety and volatile mood swings, isolation, and always loneliness.

The second dimension to illness, the second side of the sword if you will, are the social and cultural burdens the sufferer must face. In our culture, the more accepted forms of illness such as a heart attack, a burst appendix, or an attack of influenza call forth support from family, friends, and one's boss, as they have always done in the name of humanity. But the less-accepted forms, such as cancer, many of the chronic illnesses associated with the immune system, and of course, AIDS--the twentieth-century form of the plague--ostracize the patient and brand him or her as "unclean," something to be shunned and put away out of sight. After the first wave of sympathetic understanding, patients who come down with an "unacceptable" disease soon find themselves thrown back on their own resources as their loved ones get impatient, or even revolted, and return to their own lives. Relationships often crack under the stress and marriages, more often than not, break up. It is only the stablest and most loving of marriages that can sustain the burden of such illnesses. Most do not. And it is not just the emotional burdens that break people. Given the outlandish cost of medical care in this country and the woefully inadequate availability of health insurance, a prolonged illness also destroys the economic foundation of most families. And if the ill person can no longer work or take care of his or her family, you have disaster.

The third major demon ill people have to face, and which is peculiar to late twentieth-century America, is the medical profession and the American health-care system. I first became ill in July of 1984, and I was not diagnosed until November of 1985. That year and a half was devastating for me, and I now think, for the most part, needlessly so. In my search for answers, I consulted with some twenty doctors, including a trip to the Mayo Clinic. Some of these men (I came across only one woman doctor, peripherally, at the Mayo Clinic) were sincerely interested and concerned, and expressed their honest frustration as they admitted they did not know. But they were in the minority. Most of them guessed, refused to tell me anything, strung me along with vague diagnoses, or threw the responsibility back on me, a classic case of blaming the victim. As far as this latter group was concerned, since I had no clinically quantifiable evidence of disease, in their opinion I was not organically ill. It was that simple.

This either/or kind of thinking is a product of our technological age and it appears physicians are particularly susceptible. The astounding advances in technology over the past twenty years have enabled the medical profession to make sophisticated diagnoses, often non-invasively, that would have astounded our great-grandparents. But these advances are not without their dangers. More and more, as medicine deifies technology and comes to rely on it exclusively in diagnoses, individual doctors listen less and less to the patient. Just because the lab tests that we had then could not define my illness did not mean I had no physical illness; it meant we did not have the lab tests that could identify my illness at that particular point in time. While this conclusion may seem logical and obvious, it was not so to many of my doctors.

The medical profession has increasingly come under attack in the past few years for greed, arrogance, insensitivity, racial and sexist bias, and even for downright incompetence. As so many recent exposés in the media suggest, many health-care workers are compassionate and loyal to their Hippocratic oath, but an increasing number are not. Perhaps it is time to re-evaluate our cultural attitudes towards the practice and practitioners of medicine, to demystify this sacred religion, and to make accessible to all of us the truly healing touch originally associated with this great profession.

In the course of my struggles for a diagnosis of lupus and in the years since of living with chronic disease, I have encountered all of the above described problems in varying degrees. Much has been said about them in the scholarly-sociological literature, but most such discussions are inaccessible to the average reader. I have recounted my story, in part, to challenge current attitudes within the health-care profession, but more generally, to offer my experience as a general illustration of what it is to be caught up in the crucible of serious illness, in this day and time.

THE THREE-EDGED SWORD

I have changed the names and descriptions of the people involved, and in some cases, I have collapsed two individuals into one. In addition, I have deliberately omitted the names of specific locales and institutions, except for that of the Mayo Clinic, which is explained in the "Afterword." Otherwise, this account is as accurate as memory serves.

CHAPTER ONE

JULY, 1984

My problems first began early in July of 1984 with a lingering headache and a sore, stiff neck. At first I tried to ignore the pain, assuming it would go away on its own as most aches and pains of middle age do; but this episode was persistent. I noticed it most when I was driving because it was difficult to turn my head to glance at the traffic coming from behind; and not being used to using my mirrors, driving hurt. In response to the pain, I started to develop strategies to avoid the sharp burning sensation in the muscles on the right side of my neck whenever I moved my head. I made myself use the mirrors in my car. I held my head rigid, and I learned to slide off the bed in the morning instead of lifting myself up with my back and neck muscles, the way we all normally do.

Then, just as I was thinking about going to a doctor, the mother of a colleague/friend of mine died in a small town in the Texas panhandle, north of Amarillo. She was eighty-six, had been ill for over ten years, and had been dying by inches; consequently, the news was not unexpected. My friend, David, was travelling in Europe, so the funeral was delayed until he could fly home. After a couple of trans-Atlantic phone calls, we arranged that I would drive to Amarillo with a mutual friend, Irene, who had just retired from the English Department of the medium-sized West Texas university where we all taught. We would meet him at the airport in two days time; then, all three of us would drive to his home town from there.

Since I was teaching summer school, I hurriedly made arrangements to have my classes covered and tried to push aside the nagging headache and the increasing pain in my neck muscles that had been plaguing me for the past ten days. The drive to Amarillo was a trial. I held my head as still as I could, but the movement of the car, especially braking, would send the now familiar wash of pain down my neck and shoulders. I could do nothing about the situation, however, so I gritted my teeth and endured.

By the time Irene and I got to the Amarillo airport, the pain was much worse. I managed to get through the next three days by a sheer effort of will as I found out what it is like to bury someone in a small Baptist town. The wake, the funeral and the burial were highly ritualized by custom and ceremony in which the whole town participated. The day of the funeral was scorchingly hot, and as we went through the obligatory church luncheon, final visitation at the funeral parlor, and the service itself in the church next door, I began to feel really sick. Burying someone is never a pleasant experience, but coupled with the terrible heat, which was making me nauseated, in addition to the neck pain and nagging headaches, it was a trial.

Once the church service was over, I felt weak, and had to make a concerted effort not to faint. As the funeral procession wound its way through the streets of the small town, pedestrians saluted or took off their hats in respect for the dead, a quaint and generous custom that distracted me for a time from my own ills. Thank God the graveyard services were cut short by a sudden, isolated thundershower. None of us needed to draw out the emotional farewell any longer, and I knew I was at the limits of my physical capacity to present a normal front and to be supportive. Most of the mourners then adjourned to the house of an elderly aunt to partake of the funeral-baked meats, where the chatting and cool drinks somewhat relieved my emotional tension.

Around seven in the evening, David decided he wanted to return briefly to the cemetery to see the flowers on the grave, so I reluctantly went with him. The cemetery was typical of small towns. It was small, just outside the town limits, and its entrance was marked by an iron grail archway. This particular cemetery was on a hill and afforded a sweeping view of the town in one direction and the Texas panhandle plains on the other. The rain had freshened the air, and the heat of the day had somewhat diminished as we approached the grave site. The florist had carefully placed the flower arrangements on the mound of new earth with the spray of red roses that had draped the casket occupying the central position. Overcome with a surge of primeval aching that I always feel in the presence of death, I lifted my head to take in the sunset, which was incongruously glorious that evening as it spread across the West Texas sky, and once again the pain swept down the back of my neck in a sickening wave. Mustering a supreme effort, I pushed it aside and tried to offer David whatever comfort I could. We wandered slowly among the tombstones as we made our way back to the car, David pointing out to me the graves of his ancestors and close relatives on the way, a scene right out of *Our Town*. I tried to be supportive and interested, but I had had enough of death for one day, and this visible extension of it through generations made me shudder with dread. I was now thoroughly nauseated, so I gently edged us both away from this morbid scene and the stark reminders of our mortality.

Unfortunately, we were staying in the family house, which had been severely neglected during the years David's mother was gradually dying. The building itself was in disrepair, most of the trees surrounding it were dead, and the yard was full of knee-high grass and weeds. Once again, my literary background supplied me with the natural allusion--"'The Fall of the House of Usher,'" I muttered to myself, "Larry McMurtry style." And the town was just as bad. The depressed oil and farming economy of the early 1980's had hit this town particularly hard and had driven all but the most faithful to greener pastures. In the town square, some twenty shops were boarded up, leaving only the drug store, the florist, and the dry goods store to service the few people who were left.

That night, as I slept fitfully in that old house in that dying town, I was startled awake by a gust of sickly sweet, hot air that wavered through my room. David's mother, in death, had come for one last look through her house. Terrified, I sat up and read for most of the night. By the next morning, the neck pain had spawned severe headaches, and I was really beginning to feel ill. Irene and I, however, had agreed to stay a couple of days to help clean out the house, so I tried to swallow my pain and dug in to the distasteful work. I was not very successful because the neck pain was now continual, not just sparked by movement, and the headaches kept me constantly nauseated. As the pain demanded more and more of my attention, it became difficult to shove it aside and to dismiss it as nothing. Yet that is exactly what I did.

Two days later, in the late afternoon, Irene and I drove David to the Amarillo airport to send him back to Europe and then checked in to the local Holiday Inn. Infinitely relieved to be free of the tensions that always seem to surround a scene of death, in this case rendered more poignant by the dying town and that decaying house, I fell into bed exhausted. I was asleep immediately.

When we left for home the next morning, the pain was as insistent as ever, but I said little about it, because I had now convinced myself that it was tension. I had done some calculating and had decided that the upset of the death and funeral had only added to the strain I was already experiencing over some rather upsetting political events that had occurred at the university early in June. I had been the Director of Composition for the previous four years, and it had not been an easy time. Apart from the usual hassles of running a large composition program at a state university, I was constantly fighting the higher administration (who believed, irrationally, that we were doing a miserable job of teaching our freshmen to write), and my chairman, who was trying to run the department like boot camp. My term as Director of Composition was up that spring semester, and I was under pressure to accept the job for another three years. It was a thankless position, involving hours of my time, tedious administrative detail work, and no extra money.

In spite of the drawbacks, I had enjoyed the work and I was good at it. I was even willing to do it again; however, I had stipulated to my Composition Committee, which was made up of colleagues the rest of the department had elected to serve for a three-year term, that I would only accept a reappointment if it involved some kind of a salary increment. They met at the beginning of June and decided to recommend someone else to the position. I still believe that my stand was appropriate and that I deserved the raise. I miscalculated, however, in believing that I was indispensable, a common mistake we all make when we become too impressed with our self-importance. It did not take me long to find out how very well they could do without me. The resulting blow to my ego was a strong one, and the incident taught me a well-deserved lesson in university politics. Even though I have since intellectualized the experience, and I now see, with some chagrin, that I set myself up beautifully, I was terribly upset at the time.

Consequently, the first symptoms of pain that occurred early that July I dismissed as tension. I had been sitting in my back yard one evening musing on the transitoriness of academic power when I decided I needed a glass of wine to help my philosophizing. I turned my head to the right in preparation to standing up and a surge of pain, like a charge of electricity, shot down from the base of my skull on the right side of my neck to my right shoulder. I immediately assumed the pain was caused by my overly-emotional reaction to the administrative decision, and I did not, even for a minute, seriously entertain the notion that I might be genuinely physically ill. On the contrary, I was shocked at what I perceived I had managed to do to myself, and went to bed resolving to get on top of my emotions. In the following days, I consciously tried to relax in order to get rid of the pain, but it continued.

Now that the funeral was over and we were on our way home, I had every confidence that the pain would disappear in time and that I would soon be well, as had always happened in the past. I was young enough to be arrogant about my health and foolish enough to believe in my immortality. Besides, I repeated to myself, I was not really sick. I still believed, a full two weeks after the onset of my symptoms, that I had no right to feel the way I did when the cause was, after all, emotional. I had quite successfully invalidated my own experience and blamed myself, before I even approached the medical profession. I suspect this behavior is peculiar to women. Most of the men I know scream loudly and insistently when they are sick, refusing absolutely to entertain the notion that their ills are emotionally induced. And they are usually believed. Women are not, as I well knew, and in order to spare myself the humiliation of being labeled hysterical by my doctor, I did it to myself.

By the time I got home from the panhandle, I began to have doubts. The pain was increasing, and the headaches were becoming worse. It would start in the morning at the base of my neck and during the course of the day would travel up the back of my neck and skull and across the left side of my head to the left temple. I was teaching summer school and I can remember the greatest problem was trying to write on the blackboard. It hurt to rock my head back in order to see the board and I would have to hold the back of my head with my hand in order to look up. Slowly I began to realize that this time the pain was not going away on its own. It had become intense and persistent enough finally to get my attention and to force me to do what you are supposed to do when ill: see a doctor.

I made an appointment with an orthopedic surgeon friend of mine, a Dr. Lawrence Parks, whom I had been seeing for years about my back. He was also from Toronto (my home town), and we had become friends, mainly because of our shared cultural background, but also because we liked each other. I went to him rather than my internist because of my history of disc problems with my back. I suspected that I just could have a repeat of the problem, only this time in my neck. Medicine has become so specialized in the United States that it is now necessary to partially diagnose yourself before going to the doctor, so you know which one to go to. Unfortunately, this action often prejudices the situation, since the patient is liable to describe his or her symptoms to fit the doctor's specialty, and he is liable, in turn, to interpret them according to his biases. This is exactly what happened, even though we both acted in the best of good faith.

The orthopedic group Larry worked with included about ten doctors. They had their own building not far from the university, a nice structure, single story, adobe, with a Spanish tile roof. The front waiting room was large but tastefully decorated in shades of blue and green and white with rose accents. The furniture consisted of comfortable, dark-blue easy-chairs, about fifty, placed in convenient groupings, although those chairs were murder if you had back problems. I don't know why orthopedic surgeons do that, but they do. On the whole, however, that waiting room was one of the most patient-oriented I had yet experienced in my dealings with doctors. Patients registered at the main desk in this waiting room, and then were led to the various sub-waiting rooms adjacent to the particular examining rooms and office each surgeon occupied as his own territory. They all shared such facilities as clerical work space, storage, meeting rooms, cast room, and physical therapy.

In addition to being a friend, Larry had an excellent reputation as a surgeon, so I felt confident going to him. I had not seen him in a while because my back had not been giving me trouble; consequently, when he came into the examining room, we first chatted before he asked me what he could do for me. As I described my symptoms to him, I told him I didn't know if my problem fell in his area of expertise, but at least I wanted to start with him. Little did I know he was indeed only a start. He mumbled for a few seconds, and then decided, yes, it could be a cervical disc. He gave me some anti-inflammatory drug samples, a soft cervical collar which he insisted I put on immediately, led me down the hall to the physical therapy area, introduced me to one of the therapists, gave her some orders, and left.

The therapist was young and pleasant. She immediately gave me a lecture about wearing the cervical collar, telling me it was easy to get dependent on such devices, and the goal was to wean me away from it as soon as possible. My first reaction was guilt; then I was put off. I had only had the blasted thing for three minutes and here I was getting lectured about it already. Besides, I didn't want to wear it in the first place. It made me feel self-conscious, and it was hot. But she had done her damage. Whenever I put it on in the future, I felt I was giving in, and often endured pain beyond what I should have, so I would not become "dependent."

After this interchange, the therapist gave me a cotton hospital gown and told me to follow her into one of the curtained areas at the back of the room. I took off my blouse, put on the gown, and lay down on the treatment table. Then she put a compress of hot towels around my neck, slipped under my chin a leather strap which was attached to machinery behind my head, and turned on a switch. The strap began alternately to pull up on my head and then release, thirty times a minute. Then she put a stool under my knees, turned off the light and left. I felt silly. I was afraid Larry would come back and find me in this twentieth-century version of the rack and in this ridiculous position; he did. He disapproved and took me to another cubicle where he hung weights off my head down the back of the table. I was not at all sure his variation was an improvement and was about to say so, when he informed me he had to go to the hospital; some man had just broken his back. "Don't you dare go and leave me like this," I protested, to which he smiled, waved, and left, again. I endured this torture for a full half-hour before the therapist finally released me and let me go home.

I went every day for a week or so and endured sundry methods of having my neck stretched by one mechanical device or other. I sincerely wanted to get better, and believed that this treatment would help. I got steadily worse. After each session, the headaches would pound all the way home, my muscles outraged at the insult they had suffered. We finally gave up, and worried now that something was wrong with my brain, Larry insisted I see my internist, Dr. Bill Collins. When I called to make the appointment, the secretary told me that Bill (we had also become friends over the years that I had been seeing him for various minor ailments) was out of town, but that his partner, Dr. Butler, would see me that afternoon. I had not had very much to do with Dr. Butler in the years I had been going to Bill, and what little contact I did have did not particularly impress me. He did not strike me as all that knowledgeable, and had a rather bland personality. I did not want to see him, but I had no choice as the third partner was off for the afternoon. So I went, reluctantly. Butler gave me a cursory examination. He simply looked in my eyes and ears, took my blood pressure, listened to my chest, and then pronounced me fit. He did, however, take some blood, "just to check," he vaguely told me. I went home, called Larry and reported to him that Butler had found nothing wrong with me. He responded with the best of doctor clichés: "Take some aspirin over the weekend and call me on Monday."

It was a miserable weekend. By Monday, the pain was so intense that even the simple act of walking would jar my head and cause shooting pain in my neck and shoulders. My skull felt like it was swollen and I had curious sensations of hollowness and echoing in my head. The headaches were blinding and no longer bearable. There was no way I could go in to work. When I called Larry about ten a.m., he decided it was time to go to the hospital; I checked in to the one closest to the university one hour later.

I am no stranger to hospitals. I had suspected rheumatic fever as a child and had spent ten days in the children's ward of St. Joseph's Hospital in Toronto when I was seven years old. Then, as a teenager and a young adult, I had two angiograms, seven years apart, at St. Michael's Hospital in Toronto, for a congenital heart defect that turned out to be benign. Since coming to Texas in 1970, I had been hospitalized several times for female problems, and most recently for a bad disc problem in my lower back a year and a half previously. Consequently, the rituals of being institutionalized in the admissions department and then cast into the patient role once one got upstairs and surrendered one's clothes and freedom to the nurses on the ward, were not new to me. But I still did not like the procedure. I always brought my own night clothes, housecoat, and slippers, and only resorted to a hospital gown when absolutely forced to do so. I also tried to bring something with me from home, like my radio, or my favorite afghan, that I could cling to as my own. Silly perhaps, but like King Lear, I needed at least one of my hundred knights.

This time, I could not get a private room, a matter that always distresses me. When I am sick, I despise sharing the intimacies of the sick role with another person. It is bad enough for the nurses to invade my person and privacy without having a witness. Nor did I particularly enjoy overhearing and overseeing other peoples' vulnerability, listening to their television, or coping with their family. I put in a request for a transfer as soon as a private room was available, and gulped down my disappointment.

The room was not as bad as I had expected. At least it was large enough to hold the two beds comfortably, with some space left to maneuver. My roommate was cheerful enough, recovering from a mylogram (dye in the spinal column to detect a slipped or ruptured disc on x-rays), but she watched television constantly and chain smoked. I could feel myself starting to get upset at what the noise and the smoke would do to my headaches and nausea, but the nurses told me there was nowhere else for me to go. I didn't believe them. Not being an assertive person, however, I did not demand my rights. Besides, it would only be for a day, at the most, I told myself.

The nurse who came in to take my medical history, part of the admission procedure, was officious. Once you are in the hospital, any status you have in terms of your profession, or education, or accomplishments in the real world, are lost. You are now a patient, and in that role, you are defined and later identified not in terms of what you do, but of your illness or complaint--the notorious liver in 326-B. It is a humbling and humiliating experience, one that does not sit easier with use.

This dehumanization process has been the subject of much analysis and debate among medical sociologists over the years. Indeed, one has only to glance over the index to the *Journal of the American Medical Association, The New England Journal of Medicine*, or to go through the card catalogue of any library to see the proliferation of articles and books on pleas for treating the patient as a person. [1] Some analysts suggest a degree of depersonalization must exist if medical workers are to achieve scientific objectivity. Of more dubious value are the excuses of efficiency, or depersonalization as an unavoidable adjunct to being institutionalized. All, however, agree that most medical workers go along with depersonalization practices, not out of viciousness or as part of a conspiracy, but merely because it makes their jobs easier.

Whatever the motivations, the methods are evident to any observant patient. Shelley Taylor lists four major ones, beginning with what she calls routinization of procedures.[2] The hospital admitting clerk treats the anxious incoming patient as one more encounter in an ordinary working day while she asks about address, insurance, next of kin, and religion. When the patient is ushered to her room, she is routinely deprived of her clothes and valuables, and her normal individuating characteristics such as job, relationships, hobbies, are suspended and are replaced by her illness. She becomes the pneumonia case, no longer Mary Smith, Ph.D., English Professor. Deprived of her normal identifying boundaries, the patient has no choice but to accept her new diminished status as a specific medical problem to be solved in the normal course of affairs by the staff.

Secondly, points out Taylor, hospital bureaucracy depersonalizes the patient by placing him or her in a complex organization that is unfamiliar and cannot be controlled by the patient to his or her advantage. Any hospital stay will quickly teach even the most obtuse that he is at the mercy of nurses, orderlies, nursing assistants, technicians, the food staff, even the cleaning workers. The functioning of the hospital, as it has often been observed, is set up for the convenience of the staff, certainly not the patients. Contact with family and friends is limited to visiting hours, not when the patient needs companionship, telephone connection with the outside world is cut off at nine p.m., and the

[1]See Jan Howard and Anselm Strauss, eds., *Humanizing Health Care* (New York: Wiley and Sons, 1975); B. Freeman et al., "Gaps in Doctor-Patient Communication: Doctor-Patient Interaction Analysis," *Pediatric Research* (July 5, 1971): 298-311; F.J. Cook, *The Plot Against the Patient* (New Jersey: Prentice-Hall, 1967); I. S. Cooper, *The Victim is always the same* (New York: Harper and Row, 1973).

[2]See Shelly E. Taylor, "Hospital Patient Behavior: Reactance, Helplessness, or Control?" in *Interpersonal Issues in Health Care*, ed. Howard S. Friedman and M. Robin DiMatteo (New York: Academic Press, 1982), 212 ff.

patient's room is public terrain that anyone may enter whenever he or she wishes. It is almost impossible to get a good night's sleep with all the noise in the hallways, and one is awakened at seven a.m., no matter what, as the new shift comes around to take one's "vitals." On one of my hospital stays, someone, I assume a nurse, came in to my room at two a.m., wheeling in a weighing scale. She ordered me out of bed and on the scale. When I protested vigorously, she explained that they weighed patients in the middle of the night because the day shift was too busy, and the night shift had more time at their disposal. Norman Cousins tells us in his *Anatomy of an Illness*, that one of the major reasons he checked out of the hospital and into a hotel during his battle with a collagen disease was to get uninterrupted rest.[3] Nor can one come and go as one pleases. I can remember one time I presumptuously dared to go down to the hospital coffee shop with friends, and was soundly reprimanded upon my return. I have also panicked the nurses when I left my room to get some coffee from the nurses' lounge during morning rounds. "What if the doctor comes when you are out of your room?" one demanded anxiously.

A third source of depersonalization, according to Taylor, comes from interaction with the staff. They often reinforce one's status as a nonperson through simple lack of courtesy. It is common practice, especially in large teaching hospitals during rounds, for the attending physician to talk to other medical workers about the patient in the third person, in highly technical language, over his or her supine body, and to use condescending language when addressing the patient directly. Some doctors and nurses do not observe simple courtesies such as introducing themselves and thoughtlessly refer to the patient as a disembodied organ, often within earshot of the individual. The single most insulting practice, and it is done in most hospitals, is to post on the outside door of the patient's room a chart of all the liquid intake and urine output for every twenty-four hour period. Finally, deliberately keeping the patient in a state of ignorance about his or her condition and progress, while making life easier for hospital workers, contributes further to the process.[4]

A much more global study of the causes of dehumanization in health care is offered by Jack Geiger who suggests that there is a finely graded hierarchy of dehumanization in the hospital, a hierarchy which operates along racial, social and economic lines and which reflects the discriminatory processes in the larger society in which we live. He points out that "the most humanized health care in the nation is that offered to a white, (male--my addition), independently wealthy, U.S. Senator of upper class family origin, hospitalized for minor surgery at the U.S. Naval Hospital in Bethesda, Maryland, at a time when he is chairman of the Senate committee controlling appropriations for the armed forces." Then, he goes on to point out the "most dehumanized health care in the nation is that offered to a black, lower-social class, convicted criminal, perceived as politically 'radical,' or 'militant,' with a diagnosis of mental illness, in a so-called hospital for the so-called criminally insane."[5]

[3]Norman Cousins, *Anatomy of an Illness As Perceived by a Patient* (New York: W.W. Norton, 1979).

[4]Taylor, "Hospital Patient Behavior," 213.

[5]Jack H. Geiger, M.D., "The Causes of Dehumanization in Health Car and Prospects for Humanization," in Howard and Strauss, *Humanizing Health Care*, 21.

Most of us fall somewhere between these two poles and our social treatment (indeed, sometimes even medical!) depends on where our race, sex, age, social class, and economic rank places us on the status scale. I fell somewhere in the low middle, being of lower-middle income rank, female and unmarried. My Ph.D. earned me few points. Most analysts agree that whatever our affixed status, once we have entered the world of the hospital, the very nature of the beast involves some depersonalization, in spite of the good intentions of even the most caring of medical workers. The degree to which this process is intensified depends on our social categorization and the sensitivity and efforts of the staff. Some medics have jokingly wished it were possible for the patient to deposit his or her body at the hospital for repair and then to take the person home to wait.

My introduction to the above process at this particular hospital was my nurse. She cut in on the conversation I was having with Irene, who had accompanied me to the hospital, and made it clear to her she was no longer necessary. Irene left, shrugging her shoulders and huffy. My nurse then finished taking my history, crisply and dispassionately, with no attempt to communicate any human warmth. I felt sorry for the people who were experiencing their first hospitalization, frightened out of their wits as most first timers are, who had to deal with her.

I went through the rest of the admission procedure, which involved a physical exam, urinating into a cup, and handing over and cataloging all my valuables in silence. Once I was settled into bed, my nurse friend put me in neck traction similar to what I had experienced in Larry's office, ten minutes of every hour, and gave me a shot of Demerol. The drug took the edge off the pain and made me sleepy, but did little else. When I rolled over to get the shot in my hip, she exclaimed at the fact that I was wearing panties. She told me in the most condescending manner possible, "We do not wear panties in the hospital!" I wanted to point out to her that I was fourty-three years old, a college professor, I had a Ph.D., and that I did not need to be treated like a ten-year-old child; but I thought better of it. I would need her nursing care in the next few days, and I had better not make her mad at me. I reminded myself once again that as a patient, you lose your status as a functional adult and have to put up with such nonsense. Those were the rules. I simply could not afford to alienate someone who would have her degree of control over my life. But I still did not take off my panties. The woman in the bed next to me giggled.

At first I diligently followed orders with the neck traction, but once again, it only made the pain worse. Consequently, when the nurses began to slip up and to forget to put on the weights, I did not remind them. Despite the Demerol, it was difficult to turn my head, even the slightest degree, without scorching pain. The soft cervical collar helped somewhat, mainly because it restricted my head movements, but the pain was still beyond enduring. And, as I predicted, the noise of the television and the smoke from the next bed exacerbated the situation. I was awake all night with the pain, despite another shot of Demerol. I had just fallen asleep about six a.m. when Larry came charging into my room announcing himself by declaring he was not going to operate on me, no matter what. After I protested the god-awful hour, I told him I had no intentions of letting him operate on me. I was glad we were in agreement. He told me he would check with me later, and left for surgery.

Over the next couple of days, I was given a battery of tests including a bone scan of my entire body, a CAT scan of my neck, miscellaneous other x-rays, and blood tests. The bone scan was new to me. I had to lie on a wide metal table, like a tray, for over an hour, while an x-ray scanner took pictures of all my bones. I was not sure what Larry was looking for, but I trusted him, partly because he was my doctor, but more so because he was my friend. I had also never had a CAT scan, although I had seen them in use on television. The technician came to my room and gave me a shot of radioactive something or other about an hour before they took me downstairs to x-ray. Once there, he told me to lie on a metal stretcher which he then passed into the mouth of a cylindrical machine, like an iron lung. I could hear zapping sounds, "slices" he told me, as the equipment took a series of cross-section shots of my neck. None of these tests hurt, although I worried about all the radioactive material I was absorbing. Nor was I particularly worried that these tests would uncover something serious. I did not really think I had a slipped disc that would need surgery nor did it occur to me that I had a tumor in my neck or brain. Actually, I didn't even think of that one until Larry suggested it to me. I was much more concerned that the tests would show nothing, as it indeed turned out.

Part of my response was probably an instinctive denial mechanism that was working, but a much larger part was the lurking fear that maybe my pain was psychosomatic and that I had done it all to myself. In our society, having a psychosomatic illness is not a good thing to do because it smacks of malingering, of cheating and lying in order to cash in on the secondary gains associated with being ill. We humor sick people, comfort them and sympathize with them, release them from their regular responsibilities at work and at school, as long as it is determined that they have a legitimate organic illness.[6] Those people who attempt to simulate illness in order to reap some of these benefits are not tolerated and often become the focus of anger on the part of physicians who feel such patients are wasting their time. Sociologists and psychologists attempt to draw fine distinctions between psychosomatic illness and malingering, but to the ordinary person's mind, the two are pretty much interchangeable.[7] While I knew I was not malingering, or deliberately making up my symptoms for some obscure secondary gain, I certainly was concerned that my ills would prove to be psychosomatic, that is, real, but emotionally induced, and so my own fault. I was still worrying the political nonsense that had occurred at the university earlier in the summer, and I had not altogether rejected the notion that this illness had been caused by my inability to deal with the situation in a mature fashion. Further, I was afraid that if the "truth" were known, I would be perceived as being out of control and therefore "weak." I also feared that such a diagnosis would rob me of my friends and colleagues' sympathy and regard, and would bring on annoyance that I had wasted their time and energy on a "fake" illness.

While I did not articulate all these fears to myself at the time, I can now see that my singular lack of anxiety at the possibility of having cancer was an

[6]See Talcott Parsons, "Definitions of Health and Illness in the Light of American Values and Social Structure," in *Patients, Physicians, and Illness: A Sourcebook in Behavioral Science and Health*, 3rd. ed., ed. E. Gartly Jaco (New York: The Free Press, 1979), 132.

[7]See T.S. Szasz, *The Myth of Mental Illness* (New York: Hoeber-Harper, 1961), 132.

understandable reaction to my predicament. As Miriam Siegler points out in her study of the art of being a patient, it is the peculiar morality of modern medicine in the United States that it is clearly better to have a diagnosis of a terrible disease then to be accused of being a malingerer or to be told that one's ills are psychosomatic. She goes on to add that the main concern of the sick person is to have his experience of himself confirmed, hence the terrible anxiety of the patient whose tests are inconclusive.[8] While none of my test results had yet come in, my main concern was not cancer but that the lab results would not confirm my symptoms and that I would be labeled neurotic.

The second day of my stay, Larry sent a neurosurgeon, a Dr. Westlake, in to see me, still toying with the idea that there was something wrong with my brain. Dr. Westlake was in his early fifties, elegant-looking, and was thoroughly self-confident. He came into my room while I was on the phone and started talking to me immediately as he entered the room. I couldn't make any sense of what he was saying because of the other conversation going on in my ear. I broke in, told whomever it was I was talking to that I would call back, and hung up. By this time, Dr. Westlake had started examining me, and I was furious. Not only had he broken in on the middle of my phone call, he had also started to go over my body before he even introduced himself.

"Hold on a minute here," I protested; "I don't know who you are!"

Somewhat taken aback, he apologized, introduced himself, and explained that Dr. Parks (Larry) had sent him in to look at me. He performed a somewhat perfunctory neurological examination as he looked in my eyes, tested my reflexes, and asked me to count backwards. He concluded by saying he could find nothing wrong. "You are alert enough," he stated, "boy, are you alert," and left.

I suppose my feeble protest was somewhat of a Pyrrhic victory, but I was tired of health-care workers, especially doctors and nurses, walking into my room whenever they pleased without knocking, and not even observing the most common everyday courtesies they would normally afford to another human being outside the world of the hospital, such as introducing themselves and waiting respectfully for a telephone call to finish. Anyway, I never saw Dr. Westlake again, and I was moved to a private room later that afternoon, so I no longer had to deal with Nurse Panties either.

Larry dropped by a day or so later and told me that all the tests had come out negative as I had feared, except for one of the blood tests that Dr. Butler had earlier ordered. He explained it was a crude test, called a "sed rate," that measured the rate at which the sedimentation in the blood fell to the bottom of a test tube. An elevated reading (for a woman anything over twenty) indicated the presence of an infection or inflammation but was medically non-specific, which means it can be found in a large number of diseases and does not say anything much in and of itself. It does, however, indicate that something is wrong, and suggests the patient must be watched. My reading was fourty-seven.

When I asked Larry what he thought was the matter with me, he shrugged his shoulders and said, "I don't know." I was now afraid he would send me

[8]Miriam F. Siegler, *Patienthood: The Art of Being a Responsible Patient*, (New York: Macmillan, 1979), 38.

home since he could find nothing wrong, and I was not ready to go home. In addition to the neck pain and headaches, I was experiencing another phenomenon, weakness and fatigue. Usually after three or four days in bed, I get bored and restless. Not this time. I was utterly exhausted, and I felt too weak even to get up and walk down the corridor of the hospital, let alone go home. Larry, however, was sensitive to my distress because he then told me to hang around until I felt better. He also told me that he had asked Dr. Butler to further investigate the medical side of my case.

Dr. Butler checked in with me several times. On one such occasion, he suggested my problem could be allergies, and on another, the weather. It was a rainy day and he was standing in my room looking out the window with his back to me as he suggested this interesting possibility. The nurse who had accompanied him into my room rolled her eyes at the ceiling in a decided breach of professionalism, and we both mouthed "the weather!" to each other in silent exasperation. This suggestion was too much, even for her. I liked her immensely for entering into this conspiratorial relationship with me and siding with me, the patient, against the doctor, in defiance of all her training and bureaucratic instincts. We smirked at each other briefly before Dr. Butler turned around, whereupon she immediately retreated behind her professional and deferential shell. Dr. Butler then told me about the elevated sed rate and that he had checked the matter out with a hematologist (blood specialist). He assured me the test was too general to tell us anything and probably meant very little.

I languished in bed for close to ten days, during which time the intensity of the pain gradually diminished. Thank God for the summer olympics. As I hung around the hospital during that week, I felt too ill to grade the papers sent over to me from the university, to read, even to visit with my friends who dropped by. I watched every event, not just the popular gymnastics, but also the swimming, wrestling, and in desperation, archery. At times, even this activity was too much and I slept, for hours. Finally, I began to feel a little better, and one evening I turned my head without the familiar gush of pain. It seemed pointless to stay in the hospital any longer, so I went home, supposedly cured.

CHAPTER TWO

SEPTEMBER, 1984

The fall semester had not yet started, but the faculty traditionally helps out the university administration in the latter part of August with registration procedures and advising. I had been assigned to advise a group of ten incoming freshmen who had been admitted provisionally. I can remember meeting with them in a classroom of the Liberal Arts building a few days after I left the hospital, still feeling terrible. Once again, my head felt swollen and hollow, the neck pain was excruciating, and I felt nauseated and dizzy. Their poor innocent and anxious faces swam in circles around me as I tried valiantly to introduce them to the realities of university life. This incident finally convinced me that whatever had caused my debilitation, I was really sick and I needed help.

A week or so later, my internist, Bill Collins, was back in town, so I decided to check in with him. Bill was about the same age as I was, and we had known each other for some twelve years, ever since I had first come to El Paso when we were both starting our careers. He had a somewhat placid manner, although he was known to have temper tantrums, so the gossipy nurses had told me. I liked him because he reminded me of my brother. We had many friends in common, and would often run into each other at social gatherings. His practice had blossomed in the twelve years I had known him, and he was apparently making a name for himself professionally because he was now Chief of Staff at one of the local hospitals.

When Bill came in to the examining room, I recounted to him my symptoms of the past six weeks and told him I simply did not feel well. The medical profession calls this syndrome generalized malaise, which is an apt description, as I indeed felt generally lousy. After phoning Larry to check with him and after examining me, Bill put me back in the hospital that same day, three doors down from where I had been two weeks previously. One of my students worked in the admissions department, and when I presented myself to him for the second time in two weeks, he quipped, "What are you doing here again? You like the food or something?"

Bill ordered a CAT scan of my brain together with more blood tests. This CAT scan was similar to the one I had had on my neck two weeks previously, only this time they gave me an intravenous drip of iodine (contrast material, according to the official jargon) before they rolled me into the mouth of the machine. The iodine was supposed to make my brain stand out better on the x-rays. The procedure was not painful and once again I was not particularly concerned about the outcome because I did not seriously consider the possibility that there was something wrong with my brain. Many people have commented to me since that they were sure I must have been terrified by all this testing, that I was worried about cancer. But I honestly was not. As naive as it might seem, I simply did not entertain the notion that that could happen to me. Bill had told me before I checked in to the hospital that he was going to call a neurologist in on my case, a Dr. Madrid. He warned me that Dr. Madrid did not project the usual doctor ethos. "He is heavy, has a bushy red beard, and he will probably appear in your room at an outrageous hour," he cautioned. His description was accurate. Dr. Madrid first came in to my room about nine-thirty in the evening and proceeded to do a thorough neurological examination. We had just gotten started when he was called to the intensive care unit. A few minutes later a nurse stormed in, furious because he had stolen her best stethoscope and had now disappeared with it. She rummaged through his briefcase which he had left in my room, muttering uncomplimentary adjectives, then left, fuming. When he came back two hours later, I warned him about the female wrath that was about to descend on him. I was impressed when he jumped and was anxious. He was obviously not into power struggles with the nurses, and when his thoughtlessness was pointed out to him, he acknowledged it. He hurriedly got the stethoscope back to her by way of a nurse's aid, but not until after he had used it. I liked him from that moment on.

After Dr. Madrid had finished his examination, he told me he wanted to read the CAT scan before he did anything else, and if that was normal, then he would do a spinal tap, looking for possible chronic meningitis or a bacterial brain infection. He reappeared the next evening about seven-thirty and announced that the CAT scan was normal, that I did not have a brain tumor. "We were looking for something the size of a pea," he told me, "and we found nothing." The next step was the spinal tap, which was not pleasant. In this procedure, you lie on your side and curl up in a ball, shrimp-like. Then, a nurse swabs your lower back with antiseptic and covers it with a paper sheet with a square cut out of the middle. Next, the doctor injects a small amount of local anesthetic just under the skin before he pushes a larger needle into a space between two of the lumbar vertebrae below the spinal column. He then drains off a quantity of spinal fluid into a vial through the needle. The procedure takes some skill as the needle must be placed accurately. The nurse had warned me some doctors try two or three times before they get it right. Dr. Madrid did it well and swiftly, but it still hurt, a lot, and hurt even more after he finished. Further, the puncture and drainage of the spinal fluid aggravated the headaches, as Dr. Madrid warned me they would.

By this time I had been so sufficiently mauled by doctors and tests and hospital routine that I was short on patience and close to tears. Dr. Madrid was decent; it was the cumulative effect that did me in. I called a colleague/friend of mine, told him my predicament, and good person that he was, he drove immediately to the hospital and stayed and watched television with me for the rest of the evening. Really good friends know when you need to talk and when you merely need the bodily presence of someone you care about in the room. He was just such a friend.

A nurse came by first thing in the morning and told me the results of the spinal tap were normal. I was almost disappointed.

The news did nothing for my headaches, however, and they got worse during that day. I kept the window curtain closed, not being able to stand the light in the room, and I sent my visitors away as soon as I decently could. By eight p.m. I simply could not deal with the pain any more and called the nurses' station. A nurse would be down with some medication soon, I was told. Nine p.m. came, and then ten, so I called again. Same response. In the meantime, I realized the man in the next room was dying because his relatives gathered outside the door to my room and talked about it in hushed whispers. I could also hear equipment being rolled around and the beeping of a heart monitor. Trying to be the "good" patient, I waited until eleven p.m. before I called again. This time the nurses were on report, which means they were being briefed before they began their shift. Could I wait? I tried again at eleven-thirty, and they cut me off the intercom. It was not until midnight that a very apologetic Japanese nurse came in with a handful of pills. Almost hysterical from the pain and frustration, I asked her what they were. She evasively said they were to help the pain. They were also sleeping pills and tranquilizers, I later learned, the hospital's way of dealing with a "difficult" patient.

I recounted my story to Bill Collins when he came by the following morning. Apparently he read the riot act to the nurses, because the head nurse appeared in my room about noon with a cup full of Darvocet pills, which she left beside my bed. She told me to take one every four hours if I needed it, and to let her know before I ran out that I needed more. She also told me that all the nurses on the floor had just come from an hour-long meeting and that I was the subject of most of it. She did not elaborate any further, nor did I ask. Now I was worried about the afternoon shift, that they would really do me in when they also got chewed out, so I reduced my requests to a bare minimum for the remainder of the day. Yes, doctors can stand up for your rights, but they are only on the floor a few minutes of the day; one has to live with, and depend on, the nurses for the rest of the time, and it is the foolish patient who alienates them, as I had managed to do. Once four o'clock came and that same afternoon shift was back on duty, I began to feel terribly alone and isolated. I was almost frightened. Thank God I was not completely bedridden and could do most things for myself, because I did not see one nurse for the remainder of the day. I am sure they would have come were I really in need, but they would give me nothing extra. My punishment amounted to a good dose of solitary confinement.

By the end of the day, I began to feel I was the one who had been in the wrong, that I had made excessive and unreasonable and selfish demands on these people who were terribly busy with a dying patient. I had to talk long and hard to myself on the matter, reasoning that any well-run hospital should be able to accommodate the needs of a dying patient without neglecting everyone else on the floor, and that I was perfectly within my rights. Such reasonings struck a hollow note, however, when I contemplated the reality of my patient status. I was not in a position of power; they were. And if I wanted the help and companionship of the staff, I would have to conform to accepted patterns of behavior--which I had not done. By nine p.m., I was really miserable, wavering between guilt and indignation, each one canceling out the other.

Apparently, my confused and conflicting reactions were not all that unusual, according to a study conducted by Daisy Tagliacozzo and Hans

Mauksch. In their research, the authors interviewed patients at a large Midwestern medical center and questioned them closely on their perceptions of their hospital experiences. The vast majority of patients indicated an eagerness to trust those who had charge of their care, to be seen as cooperative with their treatment and hospital routine, and expressed a desire not to appear demanding of nurses. Two-thirds of the patients interviewed admitted they had refrained from expressing their needs at least once because they felt the nurses were too busy, or rushed, or had other sicker patients to attend to.

Tagliacozzo and Mauksch speculate that the almost universal desire of the interviewed patients to be "considerate" of their caretakers was a convenient rationalization for a fear of offending the staff who could in turn withhold valuable services. Very few patients showed any inclination to voice their rights as paying consumers, and those that did expressed concern that such aggressive behavior was not without its problems. Most patients quickly learn that it is the "courageous" sick person, i.e. the one who does not complain and demand, rather than the "sissy" who does, who is valued and rewarded by the hospital staff. This belief quickly transfers to acceptance of the notion that nurses do not like "demanding" patients, and that such behavior will reap punitive measures. Rendered helpless and dependent by their illness and hospital regulations, patients find themselves in a quandary. If they voice a legitimate demand for service, be it help to the bathroom or pain medication, and should this service be slow or not forthcoming, they risk alienating the very people they need to help them should they repeat their demands and become assertive. Further, and even more serious, they cast themselves in the role of "whiner" and "complainer," a morally reprehensible position in our society.

As the researchers put it, "prevalent images of the hospital as a crisis institution, the conception that rights and demands should be governed by the seriousness of the illness and consideration for other, possibly sicker patients, makes it extremely difficult to play the consumer role, openly and without fear of criticism". In other words, they continue, the problem most patients experience stems from the dissonance between the desire to broaden their sphere of control that has been severely limited by hospital practices and an awareness that efforts at such control will bring with it practical and moral sanctions. Most patients, they conclude, are reluctant to use any of the controls which are available to them, and instead modify their behavior in order to seek the approval of others. In the light of their isolated and dependent status, such behavior modifications represent "realistic responses to institutionalized impotence."[1] Nor does it appear there is much opportunity for patient behavior to change. The structures and procedures of the modern hospital, together with staff expectations, all converge to insist that the patient be passive, trustful and docile. As Judith Lorber points out, patients usually come in to the hospital singly, without a supportive group of peers, and are on their own in learning the informal rules of the organization. The patient is then isolated in a private room, or at most a semi-private room, where no sense of community ever develops and communication with other patients is limited, if not non-existent. Also, continues Lorber, doctors and nurses deliberately limit the flow of

[1]Daisy Tagliacozzo and Hans Mauksch, "The Patient's View of the Patient's Role" in Jaco, *Patients, Physicians and Illness*, 196-200.

information to patients so they cannot argue from adequate knowledge and have no basis for criticism. Should the patient reject passive behavorial expectations and attempt to be autonomous, critical and well-informed, he does so at his peril. Often he will find no one is exclusively on his side, neither doctors nor nurses, nor even other patients who may feel their share of attention will be shortchanged. And through assertive behavior, he risks the greatest threat of all, withdrawal of personalized interaction and even fundamentally necessary care. It is no wonder that a person's legitimate assertive tendencies are not exercised in a hospital setting without conflict.[2]

I was almost relieved when Bill came into my room the next morning and announced that I could go home. But I was not happy with his verdict.

"You have nothing seriously wrong with you," he declared; "the tests have all come back negative, and the pain is simple tension."

A month earlier I would have agreed with him, but now I was not so sure. I had been under stress before in my life and had experienced tension-related aches and pains, but this was not the same. At least I knew I did not have a brain tumor, but there was still something wrong with my body and they were missing it. At this point in time, however, I could not articulate such convictions, even to myself; consequently, I accepted his judgment that there was nothing wrong with me in silence. As I sat there in that hospital bed, I felt rather foolish at having attracted all this attention, apparently needlessly, but I was also experiencing a hollowness and a sense of confusion. In spite of all these negative test results and Bill's reassurance that there was nothing wrong with me, I still did not feel well.

One of my friends and a fellow English professor came into my room after Bill had left, and when I told her the verdict, she spit out "rubbish!" in her best West Texas accent. There was nothing either one of us could do, however, so after she left for the university, I called David, who had just returned from Europe, and asked him to come and get me. He arrived an hour or so later with a lovely dress he had bought for me in Greece, beige linen, full length, with gold scroll embroidery on the front and back. The gift cheered me considerably, and as I put it on and got ready to leave, I tried to be optimistic about my future. "Maybe this gift is a premonition of good things to come," I mused. When the nurses said goodbye to us as we got in the elevator, David, glib as always, told them to never mind, we would be back. Neither one of us had any inkling of how right he was.

[2]Judith Lorber, "Good Patients and Problem Patients: Conformity and Deviance in a General Hospital," in Jaco, *Patients, Physicans and Illness*, 203 ff.

CHAPTER THREE

OCTOBER, 1984--JANUARY, 1985

The next four months were a complete disaster. I plodded through the fall semester, exhausted all the time, in chronic pain, depressed, and steadily losing weight. Rest and sleep did absolutely no good, nor did exercise. I would sometimes start the day feeling almost normal and then my strength would suddenly drain out in a gush, leaving me feeling like wet spaghetti.

Whenever I would call Bill, which was often, he would tell me once again that I was suffering from tension and that it, i.e. the pain, would go away in time. I went to see him a couple of times and he kept repeating the blood tests, with the same results. My sed rate was still elevated, and in addition, I was displaying an abnormal protein profile. Apparently, the same protein results had occurred in the hospital, but no one had told me about it. He did not elaborate about what this meant, just that it was, like the elevated sed rate, non-specific. He put me on an anti-inflammatory drug, Feldene, and told me to call him in three or four weeks. I didn't know how an anti-inflammatory drug was going to help tension, and since I did not know that the two abnormal blood tests indicated an inflammatory or possible autoimmune process was going on, I was not very conscientious about taking it. Besides, it made me nauseated. So I soon stopped. I didn't know it then, but my reaction was a common one with patients who are not given information. Apparently, noncompliance with a doctor's instructions is much more wide-spread than most of us think. Particularly when the patient is kept ignorant, as I was.

As the days dragged along, and I felt no better, I began to worry about my sanity and my emotional well-being. I began to feel guilty at not feeling well, and started to whip myself for not picking up the pieces and getting on with my life. One of my best friends fueled my paranoia by suggesting that there was nothing wrong with me that a good shrink couldn't cure. The only medical person who supported me during this time was Larry, who kept insisting that I probably had some kind of virus, like encephalitis, and that "it" would go away in time. I called him every couple of weeks, and he kept asking me if I were having personal problems. "Of course I have personal problems," I evasively told him one day. "Everyone does." I didn't dare tell him about the difficulties I had had at the university at the beginning of the summer. If I told him, I was afraid that he would agree, yes, that was the problem, and he, too, would discount my symptoms. I then began to nurse a secret fear that my vague feelings of illness and the pain really would disappear and that I would be left exposed as a self-centered hypochondriac. In other words, I found myself in the peculiar situation of denying my very real physical debilitation while at the same time hoping to God the symptoms would persist as a validation of my credibility.

My friends, for the most part, were at a loss as to how to respond to me. They were generous in helping out with my responsibilities at the university when they saw I really could not cope, and were expressive of their concern as I began losing weight and started looking obviously ill. One day I ran into a woman in a local department store who used to teach part time in the English Department and who was a friend. She was with her husband, a surgeon, and they gasped when they saw how much weight I had lost. After I recounted my story briefly to them, they invited me to brunch at their country club the following Sunday and then coffee and liqueurs back at their apartment afterward. I went, innocently, had a mildly good time, and got up to leave when the other guests started to drift away. Adrian firmly put her hand on my shoulder, pushed me back onto the sofa, and told me to sit. Doug wanted to talk to me.

After the others had gone, he sat in the easy chair across the room from me and started to grill me on the tests I had had and the results. He absorbed the information I recounted to him and then told me he knew what the problem was. I had a bad case of "conversion hysteria," that is, I had serious unresolved problems in my life that I had repressed that were causing these symptoms. I very much needed a psychiatrist--"stay away from those psychologist people," he warned--and he would find one for me. I was not angry because I could see he was honestly trying to help. As he sat there articulating and reinforcing all my secret fears, I nervously unscrewed the bolts from the right hand corner of the top of his coffee table. Adrian sat beside him, grimly nodding her head in agreement. Apparently, they had agreed to initiate this painful conversation, supposedly for my own good. Depressed, I left them, wandered down to my car, went home and cried.

One of the few bright spots in my life that fall was the entry of Larry's wife and son into my life. Stephen was seventeen, an immensely likable teenager, and a thoroughly nice person. But he couldn't write. He had had health problems that had interfered with his school work, and he was not doing well in high school. Larry asked me if I would work with him, and I agreed. Perhaps if I took on someone else's problems, I would forget some of my own.

Stephen came to my office at the university every week and I found immense satisfaction in watching him grow and develop. He had a great deal of native intelligence and sincerely wanted to learn. The more we worked together, and the more attached we got to each other, the more I realized that he was a really unique person. Most seventeen-year-old kids are still ego-centered, but Stephen constantly amazed me with his interest in others' problems outside himself, and his sensitivity to my illness. We saw a great deal of each other, and as he slowly began to improve his writing and his grades, we grew to like each other very much. He did me far more good than all the doctors and tests I had so far undergone, just by being a decent human being.

Stephen's mother and I also became close friend as we conferred over his progress. Ruth was exactly the same age as I was, and we shared many cultural ties as we both had grown up in Toronto at the same time, although we did not know each other then. She was pretty and young-looking for her age, blonde and slight, and always beautifully dressed. Further, she picked up on my physical problems immediately and was a source of constant support and practical help over the next months. We liked each other immensely, one of those rare friendships where there is instant communication and mutual regard. Indeed, it was not just Ruth or Stephen, but the entire Parks family who sustained me through those horrible seventeen months, and even though I now look back on it as one of the bleakest times in my life, I remind myself that I have their friendship to show for it.

By the beginning of December, I had lost thirty pounds and apart from Stephen, any interest in my job or life. He appeared in my office one day a couple of weeks just before Christmas, grinning like a Cheshire cat, carrying a huge silver box tied with a large scarlet ribbon and bow. Inside was a lovely, and obviously expensive, silver and purple knit suit from one of the more exclusive women's shops in town. I almost cried at the sincere gesture of friendship and gratitude that I knew went behind the gift, not just from Stephen, but also from his mother and father. As down as I was on myself, I really needed that reinforcement of my value. Stephen was pleased at my reaction.

The gift did not make me feel any better physically, however. The intensity of my suffering was certainly less than it had been in July and August, but I still did not feel well, by any stretch of the imagination. I was nauseated all the time and my body felt like a dead weight. The headaches and neck pain were relentless, draining, and thoroughly debilitating. I finally called Bill again in mid-December and pleaded with him to do something. Probably to get me off his back as much as anything, he suggested I see another neurologist, who was also a psychiatrist as I later learned, a Dr. David Silverman.

When I called Dr. Silverman's secretary to make the appointment, she told me it would be weeks and weeks before I could see the doctor. However, he often made exceptions for Dr. Collins' patients. She would talk to him and call me back. She did, a few hours later, and told me I could see Dr. Silverman that same week. Now, subtly, I was in his debt, and just as subtly was handed the message that he was a busy and important person. I said nothing, however, and made note of the appointment, December 18 at nine a.m.

The waiting room in Dr. Silverman's office was spartan, furnished with cheap, uncomfortable furniture, the walls covered with some twenty-five photostated copies of various awards, diplomas, and degrees he had gathered over the years. As I sat there waiting, I wondered what kind of a doctor would frame and hang photostat copies of his credentials, rather than the originals. I was suspicious and uneasy before I had even met the man. When I was ushered in to his personal office by his nurse after about a fifteen-minute wait, he immediately confirmed my fears and reinforced the persona that had already been indirectly communicated to me. It would color the rest of the time we worked together, and it would also effectively block any real communication between us. He was a short, stocky, officious person and his affected importance, I was beginning to discover, was common among a certain type of doctor. If the patient bought it, it was of great value to him. He could then see the patient at his convenience, make him or her endure hours of waiting, undergo all kinds of tests unquestioningly, and accept hefty bills. I knew of one surgeon, who was not financially all that successful, who kept one hand on the door knob the entire time he was talking to his patients. I pushed aside my doubts about this man, however, by telling myself he must be a good doctor or Bill Collins would not have sent me to him. You have to trust someone, and I trusted Bill.

After a lengthy examination including a thermogram (ultraviolet pictures of my back to pinpoint pain centers) and subcutaneous electrical stimulation (electrodes with electric charges applied to those same pain centers to dispel them, which didn't work), and much humming and hawing, he told me that my problems were not psychosomatic. Instead, I had a myofascial dysfunction syndrome. In simple terms, this means an inflammation of the tissue surrounding the muscles in my neck and shoulders. Because the muscles in the neck were weakened, they couldn't hold up the weight of my head, hence the headaches. It all sounded good to me, and so I agreed to a series of shots of anesthetic and Vitamin B_{12} into the trigger points of the muscles in my shoulders and upper back. The shots, some six in number, were terribly painful, but I endured them, thinking at last I had some answers.

I left Dr. Silverman's office relieved and on a high. I drove over to the university and excitedly told my friends of my important-sounding diagnosis. Not knowing any better, they were impressed and happy for me that I seemed to be getting somewhere with this doctor. I returned to Dr. Silverman every week for more shots, because the effect only lasted three or four days. Then the pain would return. He would come back at me with renewed vigor, insisting that he could defuse the pain with the shots, and he put me on Xanax, a tranquilizer, and Endep, an anti-depresssant. I went around in a daze, constantly zonked on drugs, and often, not being physically able to stand or even sit, I would curl up in a ball on the floor or my office and sleep. Most of the time I sat at my desk in a dazed stupor.

Dr. Silverman would try one therapy and tell me to call him back in a couple of days to report in. I would dutifully call his office, sit by the phone all day so as not to miss his call, and would hear nothing. The next day I would try again and the same thing would happen. My days became a routine of doing what I had to do early in the morning that would require me to be out of my office; then I would put in a call to his office and wait. I would even take the phone off the hook when I had to go to the departmental office or to the bathroom. Finally, I would assert myself, call, and insist to his nurse that I speak to him immediately, which usually worked. He would apologize profusely and explain how terribly busy he was, and so forth, and the same thing would happen the next time I tried to call him. One day he even had the nerve to tell me he had lost my phone number as an excuse for not returning my call. His deliberately calculated busyness was beginning to get on my nerves, but I was helpless because I needed him. He was the only person who was actively doing anything to help me, and I told myself I would have to put up with his eccentricities. As I grew increasingly frustrated with Dr. Silverman's behavior toward me, I wondered if he behaved that way because I was female, because I was not more assertive and he could get away with it, or if he treated all his patients that way and they tolerated his behavior simply because he was a doctor. I suspect it was a dose of all three.

As the weeks passed by, Dr. Silverman told me he was beginning to suspect something more than simply myofascial pain. He indicated to me that I probably had a muscle disease, but when I questioned him further, he refused to tell me anything, asking me to trust him and to be patient. He indicated that it was his policy not to be more explicit in such cases, whatever he meant by that. I was insulted and angered for a number of reasons. For starters, I had hired him, as the expert, to give me information, and he was deliberately withholding it, as he said, for my own good. I can understand his reluctance to speculate on the possibility of some horrible disease and needlessly upsetting me, the patient, but I had asked him a direct question, and as a paying client, I felt I deserved a direct and honest answer. I was further insulted at the implication that I could not emotionally handle bad news, (after all, I am a middle-aged female said the cynical feminist streak in me), or that I did not have the intellectual capacity to absorb medical information. Finally, I was angry at what I perceived to be his patronizing attitude, his misguided paternalism, and his insistence that I play the role of the good patient, that of a passive recipient of his gratuitous attention.

Dr. Silverman's attitude toward me as a patient was a turning point in my odyssey. For the first time I was beginning to see the medical profession as a series of individuals, each with his or her own set of personality flaws and professional weaknesses. I was beginning to realize some doctors knew more than others, and some were better at diagnosis, or surgery, or whatever it was they did, than others. And some were better at interpersonal communication than others. Whatever their specific inadequacies, they had information and skills that I needed, and I would have to work around their human failings. There was simply no other way.

When I sat back and reflected further on Dr. Silverman's behavior, it started to make sense. If he didn't commit himself to any possibilities, then he could not later be wrong. None of us likes to be wrong, but it is particularly bad for a doctor to be wrong. Word gets around. Second, my indeterminate illness would keep me coming, which was to his financial gain. Third, the more ignorant I was, the more manageable I would be. He could do to me what he wanted without an argument and I would have to trust him in docile obedience. That would certainly make life easier for him. Also, to try to educate me would take time, and he already had made it abundantly clear that he had little of it to spare me. Then again, by not naming a specific illness, he could avoid an emotional scene, a situation no doctor likes. Actually, he probably simply didn't know. But rather than admit that up front, he salvaged his ego by stringing me along with generalities.

Perhaps the real basis of Dr. Silverman's conditioned behavior, however, was that by keeping me ignorant, he was the one with the knowledge and the power that went with it. It is a well-documented fact that the social practices surrounding the delivery of medical care in this country have given doctors an inordinate amount of power. Part of the reason lies in the stunning technological advances of this century and our excessive and absurd faith in them. Because of this technology, medical knowledge has become more specialized and more sophisticated, and those who have access to it have an automatic advantage over the rest of us--a power they are reluctant to share.[1] Most doctors refuse to do so on the pretense that we--i.e. patients--cannot handle such

[1]See Elliott A. Krause, *Power and Illness: The Political Sociology of Health and Medical Care* (New York: Elsevier, 1977), Chapter Three.

knowledge, emotionally or intellectually. There is some justification for this belief, as patients do vary in their intellectual capacity, education, and ability to handle the truth. It is when the physician treats all patients in a secretive manner that one can question his avowed humane motivations.

The problem of how much to communicate to the patient, and when, has been a subject of much debate over the years. Some doctors, in response to the sudden increase in malpractice law suits, make it a point always to tell every patient the entire truth, in the most unambiguous terms possible, irrespective of the emotional needs of the individual. While some might applaud this unvarnished honesty, we all know the destructive effects disastrous news can have on us physically. Dr. Mack Lipkin strongly argues that it is usually a practical impossibility to tell patients "the whole truth," and that those patients who insist on their right to know may be doing themselves a disservice.[2] Norman Cousins also recognizes the problems inherent in telling the whole truth, but he approaches the situation less polemically. He applauds the new consumerism that is just beginning in medicine because he strongly believes patients must begin to take more responsibility for their own care and cure. They cannot do that if they are kept in the dark about their disease and test results. But, he admits, the unvarnished truth sometimes throws the unprepared patient into a tailspin and can exacerbate the disease process. Then he asks the most legitimate question, "To what extent does the unembellished recital of a negative prognosis have the effect of a hex?" The patient, told he will die in five months, does just that. Surely, there is some compromise between absolute clinical disclosure and evasive, paternalistic secrecy. Cousins suggests physicians learn "to communicate negative information in such a way that it is received by the patient as a challenge rather than as a death sentence," a not unhappy solution.[3]

In my own situation, I know I was frustrated and needlessly frightened by Dr. Silverman's closed-mouth attitude. Nothing he could have told me was as bad as what I conjured up for myself in my anxious ignorance. I would like to think he kept me in the dark out of regard for my psychological welfare, but if this was his intention, it had the opposite effect. I only grew increasingly angry and soon identified him as the enemy, and by extension, all doctors.

In addition to controlling the flow of information, doctors also do many other things, some unwittingly, to reinforce the esoteric mystique of their profession and to protect their power. Since they stopped making house calls, arguing that they could not competently minister to the sick without the technology available in their offices, they have become remote and inaccessible, necessary adjuncts to mystification. And their offices are set up to further promote the image of power. Most arrangements, similar to those in the hospital, are for the convenience of the doctor, not the patient. I have been in some waiting rooms where twenty of us were packed into a room meant for ten, and the chairs were outrageously uncomfortable. The doctor himself enjoyed a personal office, which was plushly and comfortably furnished, twice the size of the waiting room. And we were the ones who were sick. Also, most doctors have

[2]Mack Lipkin, "On Lying to Patients," *Newsweek* (4 June, 1979): 13.

[3]Norman Cousins, *The Healing Heart: Antidotes to Panic and Helplessness* (New York: W.W. Norton, 1983), 133-34.

a staff of young women "servants" catering to their every need. Their obsequious deference to the doctor sends a clear message to every patient who walks in. Some doctors even dress their "girls" up in cutesie uniforms. The entire life of the office focuses in on him, his convenience, his comfort, his demands. It is also standard practice for some doctors to schedule three or four patients for appointments at the same time, on the assumption that their time is more valuable than ours, and that if we want access to their knowledge and skills, we will have to wait for it. We all know the power trip involved in keeping someone waiting. Finally, the language they use and the multi-syllabic Latinate terminology of medicine would intimidate even the boldest non-initiate.

In addition to these common practices in doctors' offices, the incomes they generate place them with the upper classes, economically and socially, thereby giving them an elevated social status and a unique prestige and power in our culture. We often attribute to them a depth and range of wisdom and knowledge on matters far removed from the practice of medicine. Witness the practice of placing a doctor or two on the boards of various foundations to lend weight and credibility to the endeavor. Further, since most doctors are white males, the socially dominant group in our society, the opportunities they have to practice racism, sexism, ageism, and cultural chauvinism are immense.[4] I think it can safely be concluded that no other group of people, except perhaps priests and law officers, has as much opportunity to exercise control over our lives.

As I meditated on Dr. Silverman's behavior and, by extension, that of many doctors I knew, my insights somewhat unsettled me because I now had to relinquish my naive belief that all doctors participated in a collective personality--that of the benevolent, selfless, caring healer. I had watched *Marcus Welby* with a passion in the late sixties, and not even *St. Elsewhere* had disillusioned me. God knows I had tested the benevolent hypothesis in the past and had found it wanting, but never had my romantic visions been subjected to the intense scrutiny they were now undergoing. As I gave up my sacred idols, however, I began to reap an important benefit of my new hold on reality. I was beginning to recognize that I was going to have to take some responsibility for my own health care and that scared me. I was going to have to make some decisions on my own and to do that, I was going to have to learn something about medicine and anatomy and diseases. Dr. Silverman was doing me a favor against his will.

[4]See Krause, *Power and Illness*, 100 ff.

CHAPTER FOUR

FEBRUARY, 1985--MAY, 1985

For a time in late February, Dr. Silverman gave up on me and sent me back to Bill Collins. When I reappeared in Collins' office, I could see that he, too, did not know what to do, and was sorry the problem was back in his lap. So he sent me back to Dr. Silverman. Finally, between the two of them, they decided to put me on Prednisone, a synthetic corticosteroid, to try to alleviate the symptoms. Dr. Silverman warned me that there were side effects to the drug and was once again evasive when I questioned him more closely. I returned to my office and in a conversation with one of my colleagues expressed my frustrations at his secrecy.

"Simple," she said. "Look it up in the *PDR*."

"The what?"

"The *Physicians' Desk Reference*." She explained it was a comprehensive encyclopedia of all the approved drugs on the market, each entry containing a description of the chemical compound of the drug, its side effects, indications for its use, and its interactions with other drugs. She assured me that with a good medical dictionary and some practice, I would find it a goldmine. She loaned me her copy, and as I explored it, I began to feel in charge of my life for the first time since I had become ill.

I looked up every drug I had ever taken, memorized its uses and interreactions with other drugs, and learned about a great many new diseases as I struggled with all the new words. Prednisone was indeed a powerful and dangerous drug and had many, many side effects. I learned it could cause cataracts, bone disease (osteoporosis), fluid retention (edema), convulsions, mood swings, anxiety attacks, psychosis, and on and on. I was stunned that Dr. Silverman had not explained all these possibilities to me so that I could make a more informed choice, and that when something unusual happened to my body, I would recognize it as a side effect of the drug, would not panic, and would take appropriate action. But he didn't. Anyway, I began taking the drug, and was prepared for the anxiety attacks and mood swings which I did indeed experience.

The Prednisone immediately softened the headaches and I began to get a glimmer of what it used to be like to feel well. Dr. Silverman slowly reduced the dosage from thirty mg. per day to seven mg. I was not cured, however. I was still plagued with the depression and fatigue, the weakness and soul-drenching malaise. I had started swimming laps at a local public pool in an attempt to build up my strength and energy level, but it didn't help. I cried constantly when I was alone, and could not take even the barest hint of criticism from anyone without bursting into tears. I knew my friends were becoming exasperated with me, and I didn't blame them. My negative behavior had gone on far too long for them to be tolerant, let alone sympathetic. In response, I withdrew from most social interaction, and spent a great deal of time sleeping. My days took on a routine. I would to to school in the morning, teach my classes, hold office hours, come home about one or two in the afternoon, take off my clothes and crawl back into bed. Then I would sleep until five, watch the news and then whatever mindless television program I could find. I would be asleep again by nine p.m. On the weekends, I would try to socialize at least one evening, but it was difficult, and exhausting. Finally, about mid-March, Dr. Silverman suggested a muscle biopsy. He told me that he had sent away to Europe for some special needles that eliminated the need for open surgery, and that as soon as they arrived, he would do the biopsy.

In the meantime, I had started biofeedback therapy in early January of 1985, which, as it turned out, was one of the few sensible things I did during that entire miserable sixteen months. I had called Larry in December, after my first meeting with Dr. Silverman, and had triumphantly reported my diagnosis of myofascial dysfunction syndrome. Not the most tactful person in the world, Larry had scoffed at the idea and told me that did not mean a thing. Thinking I had been had on a number of fronts, I got really upset with him and asked him, for crying out loud, if he had any better ideas. At least Dr. Silverman was actively pursuing something. Larry backed off, got on the phone the next morning to Bill Collins, called me at my office and told me he had arranged for me to start biofeedback, whatever that was. I told him I was willing to try anything. The therapist then called me and we arranged the first visit in early January, after I had returned from spending Christmas with my mother and father in Florida.

So, far, my mother and father had pretty much stayed in the background of my problems. They had been concerned when I was hospitalized that past summer, but I managed to reassure them when all my tests came out negative. I had communicated to them some of my troubles throughout the fall of 1984, but nowhere near the full truth. They were having legal problems, had just started a recreational vehicle rental franchise in Tampa, Florida that was keeping them hopping, and the rest of my family, who all lived in Toronto, were providing them with enough headaches to take up what was left of their time. I tried to minimize my problems, not wanting to add to theirs, but I was not all that successful. I have since learned they were scared witless for me, but restrained themselves because they did not want their apprehensions to exacerbate my situation. I warned them over the phone that I had lost a great deal of weight, but apparently they did not realize how much. They were shocked when I got off the plane in the Tampa airport. I threatened to turn around and go directly back home if they made a fuss. My mother made a valiant effort, but could not wholly contain herself. "My God, you are thin," she said through gritted teeth at the baggage carousel. I ignored her.

I spent most of that two-week stay in Florida sleeping and sunning on the beach. My mother and father had a condominium on Indian Rocks Beach, near

Clearwater, a magnificent expanse of pure white sand meeting a turquoise ocean at their doorstep. The serenity of the beach and the rhythmic sound of the water did much to restore my mental health, but not the physical. I still felt dizzy, and weak, and nauseated, and the screeching headaches returned. I was getting a bit of a tan and looked healthier, which pleased my mother, but I was also experiencing the return of an annoying rash on my arms, legs, and chest that had often happened in the past when I sat out in the sun. I found if I limited my time in the sun, I could tan and minimize the rash, which usually disappeared in a day or so anyway. I was grateful that my mother and father were tied up with their new business, as there was nothing they could do for me, and I did not want to be coddled and fussed over. For the most part, they are sensitive to my craving for independence, but not always.

I returned to West Texas in early January somewhat restored emotionally, but I knew I was still sick. My first biofeedback session was scheduled for the same day I arrived back home. I had some misgivings, as I knew nothing about the procedure, figuring it was a behavorial modification therapy that zapped you with electricity whenever you did or said something you shouldn't. I was pleasantly surprised. I soon learned that biofeedback is therapy that helps one control muscular tension and hence stress-related pain by consciously relaxing the various muscle groups in the body. The patient either lies down on a couch or sits in a comfortable chair and then is hooked up to machinery by sensors on the forehead and neck. This machinery gives the therapist such information as heart rate, blood pressure, skin temperature, and muscle energy in the form of electrical voltage being generated. He or she can thereby judge how tense or relaxed the patient is. In addition, the machine, through a beeping tone, gives the patient "feedback" on how relaxed the muscles are. The faster the tone, the more tense the patient. By concentrating on the tone, one learns to slow it down by gradually relaxing. The therapist sits beside the patient talking him or her down into a state of relaxation, and interprets the results to the patient at the end of the session.

At first I was not very good at relaxing, mainly because I did not wholly trust this rather unconventional approach to pain control. You were supposed to take pills to do that. Further, I was fighting the machines. They made me nervous, and the faster the tone would blip, the more tense I would get, which would make the tone blip even faster. I finally hit upon the idea of ignoring the tone and managed to relax somewhat better, but I was still fighting the whole procedure. It took me almost a year before I finally relaxed to the point where it was doing me any good. Most people learn the technique in twelve to twenty sessions. I really worked at it, determined I was not about to be the first person, ever, to flunk biofeedback, and the more I worked at it, the worse I got.

As I became more comfortable with my therapist, however, I got over my initial fears and suspicions and slowly learned to relax a bit. I found that the exercises helped me to deal somewhat with the constant headaches, but they were of much more value in helping me maintain a degree of serenity as I did battle with the medical profession. And it was to get much worse.

Not only did the biofeedback offer me some relief from the emotional as well as physical pain my illness had inflicted on me, my therapist, Dale Smith, was a godsend. He was the Director of Counseling Services at the hospital I always dealt with, in his mid-thirties, boyish in appearance, with sandy-colored hair, and he had beautiful, gracefully-delicate hands. He was confined to a motorized wheelchair, having been crippled by a diving accident in his youth. An intensely interesting and interested person, he is one of the few people I have met who really listens to what you have to say, and hears you. He also had a marvelous sense of humor, I was soon to find out. We liked each other immediately, and had it not been for his insights and support over the next few months, I would not have survived with my sanity intact. I did not know he had a degree in social work and was studying to be a clinical psychologist. I probably would have fought Larry, had I known. I went for biofeedback, not counseling, although as it turned out, it was the counseling that became the most beneficial parts of our sessions.

I saw Dale once a week in his scruffy office in the basement of the hospital. He shared the same hallway with the physical therapy department and the morgue; consequently, it was a real zoo down there. Everyone was on crutches, or walkers, had arms in casts, or was reclining under a sheet on a stretcher. Then there were the ones like me who looked normal physically, but who went to Dale for help with our pain. His office was a cubbyhole, halfway down the hall, with one tiny window high up in a wall that looked over the back alley of the hospital and the garbage bins. The room was barely big enough to hold his desk, which was considerably scuffed up from his wheelchair, the biofeedback machinery which was against one wall, and the recliner chair for his patients beside it. He also had a couple of bookcases crunched up beside the chair. There was a small reception area directly outside his office for his secretary, who watched him like a hawk, scolded when he was late or disorganized, and anticipated his every need with a motherly possessiveness.

Dale belonged to the new breed of therapists who call themselves cognitive behaviorists. They do not believe in making you dredge up painful childhood experiences in order to explain current emotional problems. Rather, they believe in identifying destructive behaviors that are contributing to whatever problem it is you have, and then eliminating those behaviors. We talked a lot about what made my headaches worse and better, and together we developed strategies to minimize them. His approach was completely appropriate for my problems. I did not need to be psychoanalyzed; I needed to be supported and believed.

In addition to the biofeedback therapy, Dale reviewed with me my progress with my doctors as well as the gradual evolution of my various symptoms. He offered me a great deal of practical advice on how to deal with the many other physical limitations my illness was inflicting on me with remarks like, "If it hurts your neck to drink out of a can, use a straw!" I spent a great deal of time in that basement office over the next year, and had it not been for Dale's help and support, I could not have coped.

As the weeks dragged by and Dr. Silverman's needles still had not arrived, depression set in with a vengeance, despite the anti-depressant medication. I was doing the bare minimum at work, I was not writing a freshman composition text I had contracted for, and my days consisted of struggling through my classes and counting the minutes until I could get home and back into bed. I was getting weaker, partly from the exhaustion of the chronic pain, partly from the drugs, and partly from not eating properly. I would go into a supermarket to buy food, but the smell was overwhelming, particularly at the delicatessen counter. The fried chicken and sausage links immediately called up the nausea, and I found even the relatively innocuous produce section revolting. Sometimes I made myself stay and buy food; sometimes I left without buying a thing. I often bought milkshakes on the way home as I could tolerate the milk and ice cream, and the cold was soothing. As the pounds continued to slip away, I would consciously make an effort to eat, but soon gave up again. My clothes no longer fit me, and I had to go out and buy an entire new wardrobe. At first I was pleased with my weight loss, but after I passed the twenty-pound mark, I was no longer attractive. I had suddenly become haggard-looking, gaunt and older.

Each morning, after the alarm rang, I would lie in bed and talk myself into getting up by mentally calculating how many hours it would be until I could be right back there. I resigned from all committee work at the university, went to no meetings or university functions unless absolutely necessary, and avoided as far as I could any kind of social gathering. I am a loner by nature, but certainly not a recluse. I felt guilty and unhappy about my aloneness, using it to reinforce an insecure fear that I was not all that likable anyway. So then I would try to socialize and would be sorry. I found it hard to follow any conversation, and would sit in someone's living room, exhausted, calculating how long it would be before I could decently go home. I could think of nothing to say, loud noises hurt, and I would leave a physical wreck. I soon found myself in a vicious cycle of pain and withdrawal and social isolation and suffocating depression which generated more pain and withdrawal, and on it went.

Ruth came by my office one day to talk about Stephen, and my attention kept drifting. I walked her down to her car after our meeting, vaguely aware of her presence, and almost forgot to say goodbye. My friends became distressed at how much weight I had lost, and were forever after me with unsolicited advice on what I should do about myself. Some suggested I was anorexic and needed to stop my starving nonsense. Others suggested cookies, and chocolate and fried anything. The most intriguing and perhaps sensible suggestion I had was from one of my female colleagues and friends who told me I should see a curandera (a Mexican medicine woman). I probably would have gotten more help from that source than I did from some of my doctors. This same friend also had her mother lighting candles and praying the rosary for me.

In addition to the headaches and neck pain, I was now suffering from an almost constant and overwhelming fatigue and muscle pain throughout my body. I could not stand for anyone to touch me because it physically hurt. One day my hairdresser rested his hands on my shoulders while he was cutting my hair and it felt like twenty-pound weights had descended. I could not stand even that light touch, and when I told him to take his hands away, they hurt, he was stunned. If anyone poked me in the back to get my attention, I hit the ceiling. In addition, I was having severe disintegration and anxiety nightmares and often woke up screaming. I can remember one particularly bad night when it seemed everytime I drifted off to sleep, I was immediately jolted awake by snarling animals, or grinning corpses. I often sat up all night, afraid to go to sleep, and if I did sleep, I kept on all the lights in my house.

Finally, in late May, I called Larry again, in desperation. I had given up on Dr. Silverman and his needles. Larry suggested I go to a special diagnostic hospital in Toronto. He would call up and see what he could do for me. Two weeks later I still had not heard from him. I had lunch, listlessly, with Ruth one day and she expressed her concern at the black circles under my eyes and my even further loss of weight. When I brought her up to date, she immediately went home and got on Larry's case. He called me that evening to tell me he had made an appointment with a neurologist in Toronto for June 18. I was thrown since I had expected to go to the diagnostic hospital. Thinking about it, I deduced the wait for a bed in this hospital to be over six months. Such is the state of medicine in Canada now that it has been socialized, although Larry did not offer this information. I didn't know what good another neurologist would do, but I thanked him and started planning a trip to Toronto.

Then, the next day, out of the blue, Dr. Silverman phoned me and told me the long-awaited needles had arrived, that he was leaving on a month-long vacation, and that he would do the biopsy when he returned in the middle of the summer. Once I got myself attuned to what he was saying, I was outraged and insisted he do it before he left. I was tired of waiting and of drifting along in a limbo-like state of uncertainty. I was also getting royally tired of doctors, of waiting for hours in their waiting rooms, of waiting for them to return my calls, of paying outrageous bills, of being patronized and insulted and generally made to feel like I was the nuisance of the century. In other words, I had had it. Dr. Silverman agreed to do the biopsy that same day. I was amazed at my own assertiveness. I don't usually behave like that.

I was supposed to go swimming with Ruth that afternoon, and when I called her to cancel out, she offered to go with me to Dr. Silverman's office. I agreed because I did not know what shape I would be in when he was finished with me, and I am glad she did. After the usual hour-long wait, a pleasant secretary ushered me in to Dr. Silverman's treatment room, told me to undress, and gave me a paper nightie to put on. Dr. Silverman soon appeared with great fanfare, oozing self-importance and determination, rolling a cart full of jars and instruments in front of him, for all the world like a modern-day Dr. Jekyll. The biopsy needles were curious instruments, one needle sheathed inside of another, the idea being to inject into the muscle, rotate the shaft of the inner needle to cut out a plug of muscle, and then to withdraw it up into the second shaft. From the looks of things, I was not sure this procedure was much of an advantage over a surgical biopsy, and I was right.

Dr. Silverman tried, eight times, to extract a piece of muscle out of my right thigh and failed miserably. Each time he drove the needle deep into the muscle, a fireball would explode in my leg. The sharp intensity of the pain was breathtaking. His nurse could not stand it and looked out the window while she kept her hand sympathetically on my other leg. Finally, he sent over to the hospital for a larger aspirator (suction tube on the end of the needle). I lay on the treatment table while one of his office workers went on the errand and reviewed my options. In spite of the excruciating pain, I decided I would let him go ahead because I wanted the procedure to succeed as much as he did. When the aspirator arrived some fourty-five minutes later, we went through the same procedure again, and he still could not extract a piece of muscle. Finally, in desperation, he threw down the infamous needles we had waited for all these months, and declared that he would have to do an open biopsy when he returned from vacation. He also said he would not charge me for the procedure he had just tried and praised me for being such a "good" patient. I limped out of his office, found Ruth downstairs outside the drugstore which was attached to the office building, and got her to drive me home. I was too stunned even to cry. She then went home and told Larry who immediately got on the phone with Bill Collins and all three of us decided it was time for the Mayo Clinic. Surely to God, if there was something wrong with me, they could find it.

CHAPTER FIVE

JUNE, 1985: THE MAYO CLINIC I

It was now early June, 1985, almost a year since I had first become ill. Larry called up to Rochester to investigate the situation for me and found that the earliest the Mayo Clinic could see me was October. If I wanted to come without an appointment, however, they would put me on a waiting list when I arrived and would see me as soon as enough cancellations occurred. And no, they would not take my name over the phone. They would do that when I got there. They estimated the waiting time to be six to seven days. I sure did not want to wait until October, so I packed my bags and flew to Rochester without an appointment, two days later

Before taking off, however, I went to Bill Collins' office and to the hospital to pick up all my medical records. Bill didn't really want to give them to me, but there was no other way to get them to Rochester. When he handed me the photo-copied material in an envelope, he pleaded with me not to go through his reports and grade his writing. This was something of a revelation to me. I had thought patients should not see their own records because it was not good for them. He didn't want me to see them because he was afraid of exposing his own inadequacies. After I got home and began going through the folder of material, I could understand his hesitation. I skipped over the lab tests and read the written reports first. I was astounded. First of all, Bill was right. They were not very well written, not just his, but all of them. But even more astounding, some of the reported facts were simply wrong. One doctor had written that I had had a history of headaches for the past ten years. I had told him *backaches*. And what most of my doctors had written in these reports was terribly obvious and superficial. I had expected them to be full of esoteric medical terminology and profound delvings into my medical condition, with a great many conclusions drawn from the medical facts. Boy, was I wrong. Most of the reports identified me by age, occupation, described my symptoms, and then just stopped. I could have written them myself. I could see no earthly reason, medical or otherwise, why I had not been given copies of this material.

When I turned to the lab results, I was even more taken aback. There was nothing mysterious or mystical about all this information. Most of it consisted of lab tests that were conducted during my hospital stay the previous summer, and were easy enough to read. I learned I did not have hepatitis, my cultures were all negative for bacteria, the urinalysis was clear, and the CAT scans were negative. The tests results I did not understand, I put aside, intending to ask some of my doctor friends to explain them to me later. There was one test, however, that disturbed me. Bill Collins had told me, in passing, that a protein blood test was abnormal, but the way he glossed over it, I assumed it was insignificant. As I leafed through the material, I found this particular test result, and it explained in graph form that I had an elevated gamma globulin in what they called a polyclonal gammopathy fashion. Underneath the graph, the pathologist explained that such findings usually occur in liver diseases, chronic inflammatory processes, and collagen and autoimmune diseases. This was the first time I had come across the terms collagen and autoimmune. Intrigued, I read as much as I could in my meager resources. By now I had acquired *Gray's Anatomy*, my medical dictionary, and *The American Medical Association Family Medical Guide*.

As I began to make more sense out of these terms and of the other information in my records, I felt thoroughly cheated. My doctors had had all this information at their disposal over these past months, information I had paid them to seek out, and they had not shared it with me fully and candidly. Yes, they had told me some of it verbally, but I had never been allowed to see the pieces of paper, to see the words written down, to meditate on them, and to absorb the information and make it my own in the way I had always learned new things--by reading and studying at my own pace and in private. I also felt strangely naked as I read through the reports and test results. Many people had had access to this intensely personal information, from my doctors, to all the nurses and aids during my two hospital stays, the technicians, whatever social worker happened by, even the young man who had transported me down to x-ray. But I had not been allowed to see it. This terrible invasion of my privacy made me feel squirmy inside, and once again angry at how vulnerable this illness had made me. I almost felt violated. Further, I was angry at myself for accepting the limited and edited communication I was given, unquestioningly, as if it were not my place to know more. I had never once challenged the practice of not showing patients their own records, figuring this secrecy was in the proper order of things. Amazed at my passivity and at all the new possibilities that were opening up to me, I resolved to learn a great deal more about all these test results, and to be more aggressive about demanding information when I returned from the Mayo Clinic. Never again would I be victimized by ignorance, especially about a subject so vital as my own body.

In the meantime, it became obvious to me that I had to do some sorting and organizing of all this material. I knew if I just handed a stack of reports and lab results to a strange doctor, he was not going to make the effort to organize them into a coherent pattern; nor could I expect him to. So I sat down at my computer, wrote up my own medical history, concentrating on the events of the past year, and included the reports and test results as supporting evidence to my commentary. Then I put all this information into a notebook, in chronological order, with the various sections indexed. When I was finished, I was pleased with the results. I had always found history-taking interviews unsatisfactory affairs because I usually forgot something and I knew my recital was often jumbled. This way, I would have my presentation organized when I faced the Mayo Clinic doctors during that all-important first interview. I made three copies of my report, two to take to the Mayo Clinic with me, and one for

Dale, which I left with his secretary the day before I left for Rochester. I felt that a more coherent picture of my medical problems would help him better to understand my situation and would help our therapy sessions when I got back. As I packed my two copies into my suitcase the evening before I left, my confidence was somewhat bolstered. At least I would not meet the experts unprepared.

I arrived in Rochester on a Tuesday evening with conflicting emotions. I felt a sense of adventure that always accompanies new experiences, but the excitement was muted by the purpose of my visit. I was not as tired from the trip as I thought I would be, my adrenalin probably supporting me, but I felt weak and the headaches were lurking. As the airport bus circled the main building of the Mayo Clinic, I saw for the first time the two-story-high statue of a naked man mounted on the front of the building with his arms outstretched as if embracing the ill of the entire world. I was immensely struck with the symbolism of the statue because of my own desperate need, even though it is, if you think about it, somewhat banal and romantic. As we drove by the main building and circled the rest of the Mayo Clinic complex, I meditated on the fact that this Lourdes-like shrine represented the best of what modern medicine had to offer and was (and still is) a beacon of hope to the thousands who turn to it as a last resort. Its great attraction, however, is technology rather than faith, its god, science. Nor was I impervious to its mystique. I also had put my trust in what I believed to be the unlimited powers of medical science, absolutely confident the Mayo Clinic doctors would find out what was the matter with me.

I checked into my hotel about four p.m., and then walked over to the clinic complex to see what was what. The main building was white, cruciform in shape, about twenty stories high, with a rotunda that looked like the entrance floor of a Wall Street skyscraper, all marble and elevators, and potted plants. Some several hundred people were in the area, some sitting in waiting sections reading or doing crossword puzzles, some milling around aimlessly, some coming and going purposefully from the banks of elevators. One area was particularly busy and when I went over to investigate, I discovered it was the cashier's office. Medical care in the United States is not free. The main reception area was off to the right, and since I still had fourty-five minutes before closing time, I decided to register.

The receptionist at the desk pleasantly gave me a questionnaire to fill out which asked general questions about my health and what, specifically, I had come for. She then took the form, told me it would be assessed immediately, and that I should have a seat in the waiting area. I was to receive that order many, many times in the next few days. About fifteen minutes later she called me back, handed me a small brown and white envelope, and told me to return the next morning to the fifteenth floor, west wing, section B where I had been assigned for the duration of my stay. When I looked more closely at the envelope on the way back to my motel, I saw my name typed on the front in dot matrix print and the number 3 630 873 just below it. I was now a computerized number. Having been warned by many people about this aspect of the Mayo Clinic experience, I vowed I would not let it get to me.

My motel was about a ten-minute walk from the clinic complex, about as far as I could manage in my weakened state. It was full of Mayo Clinic patients, true of every motel in town, I later learned, and was set up to accommodate the needs of such people. We all had long periods of waiting, even for those who came with appointments, so almost every motel had a central living room, usually near the front desk, with games tables, coffee and soft drink machines, a snack bar, and chatting areas. Every morning, the management set up a continental breakfast of coffee, doughnuts, and sweet rolls free of charge. Further, the rooms all contained small refrigerators and stoves for light cooking, as many patients spent up to a month in Rochester.

As they gathered in this living area, all the guests were willing, indeed eager, to discuss their illnesses, and most could not praise the Mayo Clinic enough. They spoke in hushed tones, awestruck, as they described how the Mayo Clinic doctors had identified their problems and saved their lives. Many were now back on their annual pilgrimage to the high priests, and those of us who were waiting to be diagnosed could not hear enough. One woman described her obscure cancer that had been found and cured, and another described how her husband's mangled ankle had been set right. It was interesting talking to these people, to hear of their personal lives and how they had been devastated by serious illness. While my friends and family were supportive of my problems, their lives had not been disrupted and they did not fully appreciate what a serious illness can do to one, emotionally as well as physically. These people did. I felt an immediate kinship and empathy with them.

In addition to the ubiquitous games tables and chatting area, this particular motel had a central courtyard in the middle of the building with all the rooms facing it, like a mini-version of the Hyatt concept. In the courtyard there were artificial plants and white, wrought-iron patio furniture, to give the illusion of openness and summer. It was a cheap motel, however, with no skylights, so it was dark and claustrophobic. Further, the pool, which was located in this inner courtyard, was constantly full of noisy children. I am sure it was a godsend to their parents, but it was not to the rest of us. Children are constitutionally incapable of being around a pool without screaming, and the noise, together with the smell of dampness and chlorine soon got to me. When I got back to the motel, I quickly retreated to the relative quiet of my room. Once there, I began to feel the depression settle in again. It took some effort to force myself to go out and find a restaurant for dinner, but I was determined I was going to face this experience like an adult. I found a small coffee shop about two blocks away and had a thoroughly mediocre Ruben sandwich. It was food, however. On the way home, I bought enough groceries for breakfast at a small store around the corner, paying an outrageous price for them, which depressed me even further.

I was really tired by the time I arrived back in my room, whereupon the depression became heavier. Now that night had come, the motel was even darker than I had anticipated. I turned on every light in the entire room, including the bathroom, in an attempt to counteract my gloominess and, remembering Norman Cousins' advice, turned to the silliest comedy on television I could find.[1] My tactics did little to alleviate the heaviness of my mood, however. I was beginning to feel terribly lonely and afraid. Here I was, actually at the Mayo Clinic, seeking help for an illness that no one could diagnose, and which

[1]Norman Cousins, *Anatomy of an Illness As Perceived by a Patient*, 40.

would not go away. This was serious business. Something was eating away at my health and was draining away my strength and vitality. Whatever it was that was attacking me could be life-threatening. I do not think I have ever felt quite so alone as I did that first night in that motel room in Rochester. The only sustaining thought was that at least tomorrow I would actually start to do something about all this mess. I finally fell asleep about two a.m., my bones and my soul aching.

The next morning, when I went back to the main building at the Mayo Clinic and upstairs to my appointed station, 15W-B, I was appalled. Hundreds of people were milling around and sitting in the huge waiting room, all with a look of dazed boredom, as if they had done nothing their whole lives but wait. One half of the waiting area was filled with close to twenty rows of maroon leather-covered, straight-backed chairs, each row twenty chairs deep, all facing a large reception area staffed by two nurses behind a long counter.

The rigidity of those rows of chairs reminded me of the arrangement of the countless classrooms I had encountered both as a student and as a teacher. With chairs in stiff rows, all facing forward to the center of authority--the teacher--school children get the idea at an early age about who has power and who does not. Those chairs in that waiting room were situated for maximum efficiency, and whoever placed them there gave no thought to the human needs or the comfort of the patient. Apart from being terribly uncomfortable as I was soon to discover, the chairs had the effect of reducing the patients to school children again as they sat in orderly rows facing the center of authority. The arrangement was not conducive to any kind of conversation except with the person immediately beside you, and effectively isolated patients from each other. I thought, wistfully, of the lovely waiting room in Larry's office with its comfortable, dark-blue, cloth-upholstered chairs arranged in thoughtful conversation groupings.

Behind the counter was a bank of computers and pneumatic tubing that sent information to the entire Mayo Clinic complex, and behind all this equipment was another bank of maybe twenty secretaries and nurses. From what I could gather, the doctors' offices went off to the right and left behind the reception area. This configuration was repeated in 15W-A, only they had their backs to us. And this area was only one tiny section of the whole complex. There were no windows in this room, situated as it was in the center of the building, which made it look dark and heavy. I later learned that all the doctors' offices were on the outside walls of the building, so they were the ones who had the windows.

Determined not to be intimidated, I went up to the desk and gave my brown and white envelope to the nurse. She handed me a clipboard with a general medical questionnaire on it, then told me to sit down and fill it out. I retreated to the first row of seats, answered the questions, handed it back to her, and sat down again. About a half hour later, I heard my name called over the microphone. When I returned to the front desk, the nurse told me that since I did not have an appointment, I would have to wait approximately two weeks for enough cancellations before I could be seen. She handed me a brochure on coming to the Mayo Clinic without an appointment and told me to go off and read it. I felt nauseated as I calculated how much the wait would cost me in hotel bills, squeaking a protest that they had told me six to seven days on the phone. Looking bored, she asked me if I wanted a priority interview. She carefully pointed out that the doctor who conducted the interview would not examine me, nor would he necessarily be the one to handle my case. After I agreed to the interview, she told me, once again, to have a seat in the waiting area. I slunk back to the corner of the room, found one of the larger leather chairs, and settled into it with the trashy novel I had brought along for just this contingency.

I was far too upset and churned up to read, however. After trying the first page some twelve or thirteen times, I gave up and amused myself by watching the other people in the waiting room. They came in all varieties and sizes, with varying stages of illnesses, everyone looking anxious and stressed. We were all sitting in that room like coiled snakes, ready to jump the instant our names were called. You could tell those who had appointments and those who didn't; those of us who had not yet started "through the clinic" were obviously more tense and jumped faster. The patients who already had started their workups were periodically called to the front desk over a microphone and were then either directed behind the counter to one of the two wings of doctors' offices or were given instructions for further testing around the clinic. I must have listened to fifty people being told how to collect a urine specimen for the next morning, or instructed to take an enema that evening in preparation for the next day's test.

I was disgusted with the lack of privacy and with the stripping of dignity as person after person was subjected to this kind of treatment within view and earshot of everyone else in the waiting room. Again and again I listened to peoples' private lives discussed openly, their physical complaints, their treatments, their finances, their family. One woman, a nun, so the nurse loudly announced, had to admit to female problems in front of us all, and an elderly and distinguished-looking judge was told to sit down and wait until he was called. I am by nature a private person, so I was super-sensitive to these peoples' humiliations. I squirmed for them, as I squirmed for myself when my turn came.

I was further struck by the tolerance of all these people, that they would let themselves be subjected to this kind of treatment, that they would place themselves, as I had, in this submissive role totally at the mercy of the Mayo Clinic staff. These were people, many of whom outside the world of this clinic were professionals, used to taking charge of their lives, and under normal circumstances never would have tolerated the waiting and the undignified scenes at the front desk. Not only that day, but throughout my entire Mayo Clinic experience and during the months that followed, I often had occasion to reflect on the behaviors of ill people and of those who treat them.

Much of the literature on the above subject points out that illness is a narcissistic insult to one's integrity, to our sense of wholeness, and is in itself a humbling experience. It explodes rather rapidly the universal and totally irrational assumption that we are capable, self-sufficient, that our bodies are indestructible, and that we can control the world around us. A sudden illness reduces us to a state of confusion and anxiety, and in this crisis state, many of us behave in totally inappropriate and childish ways as we try to bumble our way around a foreign role and a foreign environment. For medical personnel, illness is an everyday matter, nothing to get excited about, and the trappings of the health-care environment are familiar. For the patient, it is all new and mysterious. He doesn't know how to behave, or what to think, or what to do; he is an amateur in somebody else's professional world. And he is frightened. So he does what he is told to do and accepts the conventions of doctors' offices, and waiting rooms, and the appropriate patient submissiveness unquestioningly. Further, he puts his naive and total trust in his doctor and meekly accepts the subtle abuse. In the fundamentally human drive to live and to feel well, we are all willing to set aside our dignity, our independence, indeed our very identities, in return for what we think the wonders of modern medicine can do for us.

The Mayo Clinic prides itself on being efficient and cost effective. That it certainly is. But at a terrible price. I am sure every one of us in that waiting room reasoned with ourselves that if we had to be dehumanized by the invasion of privacy at the front desk, if we had to wait for hours, and to endure the controlled tension in that room, it was worth it. We needed to see these doctors, not a specific one, but any doctor, because they knew things that could help us. We could no longer help ourselves, and in the role of supplicant, we had no choice but to accept their rules. They were the only route we had to the marvels of medical technology. So we waited in those impossibly uncomfortable chairs, sitting in straight rows, and came and went when we were told.

After about two hours of sitting, the tension and the exhaustion from the trip to Rochester finally caught up with me. I began to feel nauseated again, the left side of my head began pounding, and I grew increasingly uncomfortable in those hard leather chairs. Finally, I decided it was time to find a ladies' room. I was nervous, however, that they would call me while I was out of the waiting area and that I would lose my interview. I trekked back to the main desk, explained my predicament to the nurse, who, without even looking at me, said there was a loudspeaker in the restroom.

The ladies' room around the corner was a far different place from the tense and orderly atmosphere of the waiting room. Out there, no one dared talk to each other, nor could one smoke, nor drink, nor eat; the main focus of life was to hear your name over the loudspeaker. No so here. The smoke in the air was overwhelming as the smokers inhaled and exhaled deeply. I had given up smoking several years previously, and my chronic state of nausea made even the thought of smoking a disgusting prospect. But I could certainly identify with the need of these women to relax and to cut through the high-pitched tension that existed out in the waiting room. In my entire experience at the Mayo Clinic, this was the only room where I saw patients relaxed, chatting to each other, drinking coffee, in a kind of communal sharing. Of all places, the restroom was the only place where we could be ourselves, with no clinic staff present to remind us of our infirmities and our subordinate status, where we did not have to sit in rows, where we could talk to each other and engage in personal hygiene rituals that were familiar and common. Life was pleasant here, except for the shattering intrusion of the loudspeaker that every once in a while called an individual back to the main desk immediately. I left quickly because of the smoke, but I would much rather have done my waiting in that bathroom than in the space the Mayo Clinic had designated we should wait.

About eleven-thirty, I finally heard my name. I went up to the desk and was told to come back at one-thirty. A doctor would see me as soon as one was available that afternoon. Dejected, I wandered off for lunch. It is impossible in

Rochester to get away from the Clinic patients. I had lunch at a counter in the coffee shop of the famous Kahler Hotel across the street from the main Mayo Clinic building with a gentleman who sang the praises of the clinic throughout his entire hamburger. He told me he goes to the Mayo Clinic every year for his annual checkup and warned me not be too passive during my workup. "Patients have to be aggressive and creative in their own evaluations," he stated, "and not leave everything to the doctors." I was impressed, but doubted that I could be that assertive. When I told him I was discouraged at the possible wait and that I was considering turning tail and running, he was disgusted. He told me that I was going to stay, no matter how long it took, that I was being childish and immature, went back to his hamburger, and refused to talk to me anymore.

At one-thirty, somewhat humbled by the lecture I had received at lunch, I again signed in at 15W-B and settled in for a wait. The familiar headaches, neck pain, and nausea intermittently demanded my attention as I struggled to find a comfortable position in those terrible chairs. I had been waiting for barely an hour when, to my amazement, I was called by a nurse standing at the right side of the front desk. She smiled at me, and led me into the right wing of doctors' offices. The room we finally entered doubled as an examining room and office, and, as I was to discover, was repeated hundreds of times throughout the clinic. At one end, on the right was a desk, and beside it, along the wall was a low padded bench. On the other side of the room were a sink and an examining table. Behind the table was a small curtained area where the patient dressed and undressed. Most doctors discreetly leave the room while you undress, but this was apparently not the case here.

There was not one square inch of wasted space in this office, and the furniture looked like it came from a medical supply warehouse: clean, functional, and wholly without character. On the left side of the desk was a series of pigeon holes containing colored cards that I later learned were entry slips to the various stations around the clinic where diagnostic tests were performed. This particular doctor had tried to personalize his cubby hole with pictures of seals and dolphins on the wall beside his diplomas and with a couple of bedraggled plants on the windowsill, but he was not entirely successful. The nurse told me to sit down on the bench beside the desk--which firmly placed me lower than anyone seated at that desk, I cynically observed--and that the doctor would be there shortly.

When he came in, a nondescript person of slight build in his early fifties, about five minutes later, he was efficient, like his office, as he asked me to explain myself. My major in my Ph.D. work was in rhetoric, so I immediately pulled all my skills into action. I carefully explained to him my problems, then handed him the notebook of medical records and history that I had painstakingly gathered and indexed for just such a meeting. He was impressed, and after questioning me for some thirty minutes, assigned me to the "urgent" category, which meant I was number three on the waiting list for a cancellation, instead of number thirteen. When I returned to the front desk, the nurse told me that meant I would be seen in one to three days, and that I was to come back tomorrow morning and wait.

Pleased with myself, I left the Mayo Clinic, found myself a bar, and had a drink. I was even feeling well enough to eat something, so I went for a walk, found a nice restaurant, and had a leisurely dinner. Not even the depressing atmosphere of the motel could get me down when I later returned. For the first time I felt that I was in control, if not of my illness, at least of my treatment. For once, by doing my homework and using some of my professional and interpersonal skills, I had made the medical profession behave in a manner suitable to my needs, instead of the other way around. My victory, however, was short-lived. I should have known better than to take on such a monolithic institution as the Mayo Clinic.

The next morning, I reported back to 15W-B promptly at 8:30 a.m. and once again settled in to wait. By listening to the anxious conversations at the front desk, I could gauge where I was on the waiting list. Those even more strung out than I was checked every half hour. Those without appointments were gathered every morning in case of cancellations or no shows. The nurses knew if there was to be an opening by approximately ten-thirty and called those waiting to dismiss them for the day at that time if no openings had come up. Then they were told to come back the next day and repeat the process. One or two openings a day was normal for each of the stations throughout the clinic. The brochure the nurse had given me the day before explained these last-minute openings became available because of the huge patient volume the clinic processed, which was particularly large now that the nice weather was approaching.

As I listened to the conversations at the front desk, I was amazed to discover that many people came to the Mayo Clinic for their annual checkups. One couple who had been vacationing in the area explained they had dropped by on a whim to see if they could have a checkup. One person got pushy and demanded an interview immediately, but there were few of these. Not many people assert themselves to medical personnel, even nurses, and this was, after all, *the* Mayo Clinic. The nurse on duty handled all these people with stern yet pleasant effectiveness, and there were surprisingly few temper flares, given the tense dynamics of the situation.

When I was finally called at exactly 10:45, I expected to be sent home for the day, but to my surprise, another nurse took me behind the counter, measured my height, weighed me, and led me to a doctor's office. Even more to my surprise, it was the same office I had been in the day before. The nurse smiled and told me Dr. Campbell was so impressed with my presentation that he had decided to take me on as an extra patient so that I could begin to "go through" the clinic immediately. Once again I sat down on the low bench and waited. When Dr. Campbell entered the room and I thanked him, he told me crisply that he felt I had enough symptoms to warrant immediate investigation. I silently thanked whatever star it was that had made me a rhetorician, and we began.

Dr. Campbell went over my notebook in painstaking detail and questioned me closely about every event in my medical history. I have an "interesting" congenital heart deformity that is benign and asymptomatic, a condition which caught his attention far more than my other array of vague complaints. I have lived with this heart problem all my life and it has come to bore me when doctors become excited about it. Once I got him off that topic, I felt that we were really getting somewhere with my present illness. He seemed to hear me and to take me seriously, although it was hard to read what was going on behind the professional mask that was firmly in place. He showed little interest in me as a person, only once letting his own personality emerge. As I was climbing up on the examination table in front of the window, I was struck by the lovely view. Having just come from the desert with its heat and barren landscape, I was stunned by the soft beauty and rich greenery of the Minnesota spring countryside. When I remarked on it, he smiled, but said nothing.

He was most careful with the physical examination. He went over my eyes, ears, nose, throat, looked at my scalp, tested all my reflexes, listened to my lungs and chest, prodded at my belly, felt all my glands, took my temperature, made me swallow water while he felt my thyroid. I felt humiliated by the time he had finished, as I always do when a strange doctor examines me, and try as I might, I cannot reduce it to a scientific encounter. When I emerged from his office at just after two in the afternoon, however, I felt I had gotten my money's worth. He ordered a whole battery of tests that kept me busy for the next three days. I went from department to department for blood tests, electrocardiograms, echocardiograms, x-rays, an electromyograph, and then finally, for consultations with a neurologist and a rheumatologist. This last interview somewhat unsettled me. The doctor was in his early thirties, good-looking, and as arrogant as they come. I knew his type. I have many colleagues like him, and I was suspicious. He was rough as he examined me, grabbing the muscles that I told him hurt, and squeezing them much harder than was necessary. I was thoroughly annoyed when I left his office, but soon dismissed him as an uncaring smart alec.

After I had left Dr. Campbell that first day, I was told to wait for an hour or so for my schedule of tests to come up from the computer. When they were ready, the nurse called me up to the front desk once again and proceeded to fill my brown and white envelope with a series of cards, each one for a specific test at a specific time and place. Then she gave me a computerized list of all my appointments and sent me on my way. As I chased around the clinic and submitted myself to the multitude of tests that Dr. Campbell had ordered, I slowly developed a sense of the absurd and a kind of weird sense of humor. For example, in the x-ray lab, the women went in groups of twenty to the right and the men in groups of twenty to the left. We were led to a row of small cubicles where we were told to take off our clothes, to put on the Mayo Clinic version of the examination gown (sans sleeves, like an inverted cape, two back to back if we were walking around anywhere), and to put our clothes in an assigned locker. We were then given the key to our locker which was fastened to an elastic band placed over our wrists. A nurse then led us down a hall and told us to sit on benches in the hallway. By this time I got the giggles at the absurdity of the whole situation, and visions of *1984* popped into my head. When I tried to convey my amusement to the woman next to me, she just appeared embarrassed.

Elsewhere, the patients developed a kind of gallows humor and camaraderie. In the purple blood-letting room, (there were also the green room and the yellow room) the man in front of me was as nervous as a cat. He finally blurted out that he had never endured a needle in his life. The rest of us were dumbfounded, and when his turn came, we all wished him luck. When he came out, he gave a victory sign, declared it didn't hurt, and we cheered him out of the room. I have never ceased to be amazed at the resilience of human nature, especially when we are being subjected to the humiliations of medical procedures.

I was also struck by the stoicism of many of my compatriots. Most of the patients had a family member with them to help them through the stress of the testing and the waiting and to ease them through any bad news. I would advise anyone who has to go through such an experience to bring some kind of moral support. It is really necessary. A couple of teenagers appeared to be on the same track as I was, and were obviously by themselves. Apparently, their worried parents had scraped together the money to send them to the best medical clinic in the world, but could not afford to accompany them. I was impressed with their courage and grace as they confronted what must have been a most frightening experience for them. But they, like me, were comforted by the aura of the Mayo Clinic, and put their trust in the people who were doing these things to them.

Most of the tests were conducted by technicians and while they were polite, there was little response to the patient as an individual. I am sure the sheer volume of people who passed through their hands dictated against any kind of personalization, but to their credit, some of them tried. The young resident who did the echocardiogram (a heart test using ultra sound), however, was an oaf, with absolutely no sensitivity to the modesty of his patients. He was tall, had gangly arms that hung out the ends of his too-small white coat and wore baggy pants and scruffy rubber-soled shoes. He called me out of the waiting room, told me to strip to the waist in a cubicle in the hallway, leave my clothes there, put on a gown, and then to come into the test room. I dutifully obeyed, and after I had lain down on the bed which was obviously meant for the patient, he took away my gown and hooked me up to the machinery by placing electrodes all over my chest.

After he had done his readings, he called in the head of the department and four other residents to look at this interesting case. As they all trooped in, I felt like Prufrock's fly squiggling on the end of a pin. Dr. Campbell had asked me to submit to the echocardiogram supposedly to check up on a chronic condition "while I was there." I was beginning to wonder, however, just whose interests this test was serving. I was really starting to get angry, and besides, I was long overdue for an appointment with Dr. Campbell back on 15W-B, when they decided they were finished with me an hour and a half later. The resident told me I could go back to the cubicle and dress, but he did not give me back my gown. When I pointed out that I might get arrested for indecent exposure on the way, he merely shrugged and handed me the gown.

The most pleasant contact I had with Mayo Clinic doctors was with the woman neurologist who did the muscle conduction study, called an electromyograph (EMG). The test consisted of a series of electric shocks applied to my right arm through a small needle to see if the muscles and nerves were in proper working order. The test was mildly unpleasant, and took about three quarters of an hour. I was much more interested in talking to this woman, however, because she immediately responded to me as a fellow professional, not as a patient. We chatted about where we had studied, and how we both wound up in our present jobs, and I asked her if she liked living in Rochester, and she asked me if I liked living in Texas. She was not at all condescending, and for the first time since I had come to Rochester, I was allowed to step out of the patient role and be a real human being. I felt I did not have to be on my guard with her, nor was I fighting her. The resulting release of tension was magical. We discussed my medical situation and our respective careers as one adult to another, a unique experience for me thus far in my dealings with the medical profession. I was sorry to leave her.

In addition to all the physical testing, I was also given a psychological test to take that first evening that I later understood to be the Minnesota Multiphrastic Personality Inventory (MMPI), an old standby in evaluating a patient's psychological status. This part of the workup bothered me because as I took it, I vaguely sensed something was happening that was beyond my control. As I was checking off the answers on the computer card that evening in the motel, I felt uneasy. Many of the questions I would have answered differently before I got sick. I found myself agreeing yes, I am depressed; yes, I do not sleep well at night; yes, I wake up feeling tired; yes, I am not functioning as well at work as I normally do; yes, I have chronic headaches. I worried about the profile I was creating and considered being less than truthful. I decided, however, that it was not in my best interests to play games, and completed the questionnaire as truthfully as I could. I even said yes, I have lied in my life (who has not, for crying out loud!), and yes, I have abused alcohol. I still vividly remember one New Year's Eve when I was in college in Toronto when I got thoroughly snockered on Teacher's whiskey. Nor was that an isolated incident in my youth. Trustful and naive, I cheerfully handed in my MMPI packet the next morning, and went on about my business.

CHAPTER SIX

JUNE, 1985: THE MAYO CLINIC II

I had arrived at the Mayo Clinic on Tuesday evening, had first seen Dr. Campbell on Wednesday afternoon, and had begun my workup on Thursday morning. Dr. Campbell had scheduled tests for Friday, Monday, and Tuesday, and I was to report back to him late Tuesday afternoon. That meant I had the weekend to kill. My mother and father arrived Thursday afternoon, having driven from Florida where they spend the winters, on their way up to our summer home in Canada just north of Toronto. I was dubious about their coming because they both have such strong personalities they dominate whatever situation they are in. I had already been robbed of a great deal of my adult status by this illness, and I knew their presence, albeit unwittingly, would rob me of more. Even when I am well, I feel like a little girl around them. However, I had to admit I was frightened, and having faced down the Mayo Clinic doctors for three days on my own, I was ready for some moral support.

Also, I realized they needed to come. Despite my age, I was still their progeny, and alone, and ill. The specter of the Mayo Clinic is comforting, but it also conjures up images of terrible and frightening illness, and desperation. My presence in Rochester associated with my condition an urgency and a seriousness that had not been there before. They were truly concerned and frightened for me. Also, I was sure they had felt frustrated and helpless those past months as I recounted to them my experience with my doctors back home over long-distance telephone. Coming to Rochester gave them something concrete they could do, and I owed them that. Then again, the approaching weekend looked long and empty, and I did not really want to be alone for two days with nothing to do. I knew what that would do for my depression. Finally, being really honest with myself, I decided I was grateful they were coming. As much as I hated to admit it, I wanted my mother.

My mother and father, in their late sixties at the time, were both vibrant people. My father always was, and still is, a distinguished-looking man. He is tall, has steel-gray hair, is a retired Wall Street executive, and carries with him that executive authority. A family friend once described my mother as a Miss Ellie, a comparison I found particularly apt. She is short, sensitive and motherly, but strong. Between them, they had propagated a rather large brood. I was one of five and my brothers and sister among them had managed to produce a total of twelve grandchildren. Such a large family is not without its share of problems, however, and my parents were constantly having to put out fires as they rescued whichever one of us had managed to get in trouble. I was their latest problem.

Their first action upon arriving in Rochester was to change motels. The dark atmosphere of the motel I was in was getting to me, even though it was convenient to the clinic, so I did not object. We moved to a much sunnier motel on the edge of town, and although the rooms and surroundings were nicer, I soon discovered that I had lost my mobility. I could no longer come and go on my own, having to depend on them to drive me everywhere. They were good about picking me up and dropping me off promptly, but the situation made me dependent on them, as I had anticipated it would. Once again they were in control of my life. I began to regress in age by the hour, and I soon found myself taking my usual defensive course when I feel diminished--withdrawing. In spite of all these complicated dynamics that I always experience whenever I am with my parents, this time I decided their companionship and loving concern outweighed the disadvantages. I was determined to be grateful they were there.

They spent Friday amusing themselves touring the Mayo Clinic facilities while I had tests, but I could tell they would soon get bored and restless, which made me nervous. So when I suggested we get out of Rochester for the weekend and away from old and sick people, walkers, and wheelchairs, they quickly agreed. We drove up to Minneapolis Saturday morning, checked in to a motel on the edge of town, and went shopping on the refurbished Nicollette Street. After an hour or so of window shopping and strolling, we stopped at an outdoor restaurant for a beer and a sandwich to enjoy the sun and to watch the passing parade. I gloried in the youth and health of the strutting teenagers around the streets. One girl had her face powdered white and was sporting black lipstick and nail polish; still she looked healthy. Illness had not even entered into the realm of possibility for these young people. Enjoy your good health, savor it, I whispered to them. We wandered through shops for the rest of the afternoon and then picked up tickets for a production of *Cyrano de Bergerac* which was playing at the Guthrie Theater that evening. It was long and a bit heavy for my mother and father, so we left early. I was not all that disappointed, mainly because I was feeling nauseated and exhausted from all the sightseeing. I was trying to carry on as normally as I could, but I was sick, and no amount of denial was going to make that fact go away.

The next morning, we checked out of the hotel, drove to St. Paul and explored the science museum. Then, in the late afternoon, we headed back for Rochester. Throughout this entire weekend, I was beset with strange and conflicting emotions. I was glad my mother and father were with me, and yet I resented my increasingly dependent status. I was having a good time with them, and yet I could not for a minute forget why I was in Minnesota. At one point I can remember looking in a store window at an exquisite Japanese urn, completely bound up in the beauty of the object, when I saw myself faintly reflected in the glass window. I looked terrible, thin and pasty white, and ill. I turned away from the store with a sinking feeling. This kind of experience happened often. Just as I would begin to enjoy myself, something would happen to remind me of my physical ills and jolt me back to reality. As the weekend dragged on, my headaches began to intensify, and I could hold up my head only with a great deal of difficulty. I had brought the soft cervical collar Larry had given me the past summer, but I hesitated to wear it because it made me feel self-conscious. The pain got too much, however, and I was forced to put it on. Finally, not even the collar helped. The pain on the left side of my head was building, and any movement of my left jaw sent a sharp stab up the side of my head and behind my left eyeball. I was almost glad to get back to Rochester on Sunday evening, to get on with the business of being ill. The weekend was an unnecessary distraction, off the point.

The Mayo Clinic is one of the most efficient medical facilities I have ever encountered. The number of tests and consultations, if done at home on a routine basis, would have taken weeks to set up, let alone accumulate results. By late Tuesday, I was ready to return to Dr. Campbell to confer with him on the test results and on a possible diagnosis and treatment. I gathered during the course of the various tests that they were considering several muscle diseases and one by one were ruling them out. They decided I did not have polymyositis or polymyalgia rheumatica, both inflammatory muscle diseases, because the EMG was normal and the various doctors who examined me did not find muscle weakness. The left temporal headaches, however, led them to believe that I might have giant cell arteritis, an inflammation of the arteries that often manifests itself with left temporal headaches. If left untreated, the disease can cause blindness and strokes, and unfortunately, the only way to diagnose it is to do a biopsy of the artery. When I saw Dr. Campbell again on Tuesday afternoon, he carefully explained the situation to me and recommended a left temporal artery biopsy. They could do it for me on Thursday morning on an outpatient basis at one of the hospitals affiliated with the Mayo Clinic. I agreed, and even though I did not relish the surgery, I felt we were finally getting somewhere.

Dr. Campbell arranged for me to meet with the neurosurgeon the next day (Wednesday) and to have the surgery first thing Thursday morning. I met the surgeon briefly on Wednesday, about noon, in Dr. Campbell's office, whereupon he warned me about the possibility of my eyelid drooping after the surgery. He felt the left temporal headaches were sufficiently alarming, however, to go ahead with the procedure. He was obviously an important person; everyone in the doctors' area of 15W-B deferred to him immediately. He had his nurse with him, dressed in a dark blue suit and carrying a clipboard, taking down his every order. She basked in his reflected glory, important because she worked for an important person, and kept smiling at me condescendingly. I felt like kicking her. This whole experience really was reducing me to infantilism.

When my parents picked me up that afternoon, I told them I was going to have the biopsy the next morning. They took it in stride, trusting the Mayo doctors, sure that we were finally going to come up with some answers. While I accepted the surgery as the logical next step, I was definitely not looking forward to it. I had undergone enough medical procedures in the past to understand what was involved, and I knew there would be pain and upset. They try to minimize the anxiety by assuring you there will be "discomfort," not pain, but I knew better. Dr. Silverman had also assured me his biopsy needles would not hurt.

The neurosurgeon had explained that they were going to have to shave the side of my head. Then they would give me a local anesthetic, after which they would cut out a small piece of the left temporal artery for biopsy. The whole procedure would take about three-quarters of an hour. I was apprehensive about the pain I knew would be associated with the biopsy, but also knew it would not last for long. I was more immediately concerned at the prospect of having the side of my head shaved and that I would not be able to wash my hair for a couple of weeks. I have dark-brown, naturally-curly hair and to keep the curls looking fresh and natural, I wash it every morning in the shower. My physical appearance had deteriorated enough with my illness; I could just imagine what a partially shaved head and two weeks' build-up of oil in my hair would do to me. My mother, however, came up with a solution. We went to the drugstore that evening, and she bought me some dry shampoo. Then she found a couple of long scarves that I could tie over the front part of my head covering my ears and hopefully the part of my skull they were intending to shave. One was a pink mesh and the other was purple, both matching the clothes I had brought with me to Rochester. Vanity, thy name is woman, to misquote Hamlet. I suggested to my mother that when they were finished with me, maybe I should dye my hair on the other side of my head green, and I could go punk, like the kids in Minneapolis. She was amused.

I checked in at the outpatient reception area on the main floor of the hospital at six a.m. Thursday, where a middle-aged female secretary took my insurance information and then immediately led me to the outpatient quarters on the third floor. There, I was greeted by a nun who took me into a fairly large room where she gave me a hospital gown, a seersucker housecoat, a pair of slippers, a paper surgical cap, and the key to a locker. She told me to undress in one of the cubicles that lined the side of the room. The lockers ran the length of the other side of the room. I knew she was a nun only because she introduced herself as Sister Sweeney. She was dressed in blue surgical scrubs and wore a blue surgical cap on her head, like everyone else. Times sure have changed I can remember thinking. Then she told me I could "empty my bladder" in the ladies' room off to the right. That euphemism always amuses me and it is ubiquitous among nurses. Once I was undressed, had deposited my clothes in one of the lockers, and had dutifully gone to the ladies' room, Sister Sweeney took me to an adjacent room where she told me to sit on a stool beside a counter and then took my medical history. I could by now rattle off all pertinent information in five minutes flat. Then she took my temperature and blood pressure. Besides that counter and the row of shelves above it, the room contained four or five recliner chairs where patients recovered from their surgery, so Sister Sweeney explained. It all looked quite cozy.

Then a second nurse came by, led me to a stretcher in the hall, and told me to climb on. After covering me with a sheet, she rolled me down the hall and through swinging double doors into a surgical holding area. The room was huge and dimly lit, permeated with a hushed quiet. There must have been thirty other people there, lying on stretchers lined up side by each, some out cold, some moaning, and most, like me, staring at the ceiling. We all looked the same, inert masses waiting to be cut open, nothing more.

From time to time someone would walk by, look at the name tag taped to the bottom of a stretcher, and move one. No one ever looked at our faces, or talked to us, or made any attempt at human contact. They talked to each other about us, in the third person, with such comments as "this one's not ready yet," or "this one will have to wait." The only uniqueness we had to these people was the specific procedure we were to undergo. No one attempted to reassure us or chat to pass the waiting time, or to give us any hint of human compassion. Nothing. Assembly line medicine in the extreme. It was almost a parody. We could have been bodies in a morgue for all these people appeared to care. To counteract the almost surrealistic atmosphere, I tried consciously to shut out my surroundings and deliberately to concentrate on myself so that I would not lose a sense of who I was.

"This is not going to go on forever," I told myself. "I will get out of here."

There was a brief flurry as one women two stretchers down from me started wailing and a flutter of attendants converged on her stretcher. They soon knocked her out with a shot of something or other. I lay there, rhythmically reciting to myself, "One flew east, and one flew west, / And one flew over the cuckoo's nest." Ken Kesey did know what he was talking about. To my surprise, they gave me nothing, no relaxant, not even aspirin.

Finally, a white-garbed attendant stopped at my stretcher, checked my number taped on the bottom rail against a chart on the clipboard he held in his hand, and wheeled me out of that awful room. We went down halls and around corners, and he left me in a hallway outside the operating room where I was apparently assigned. The hallway ran along the outside wall of the building which was covered with windows that faced a lovely park area. As I lay there gazing on the scenery from my stretcher, once again I was struck with the emerald green of an upper-midwestern spring. The beauty of the landscape, instead of soothing me, however, made me feel terribly lonely and sad. Serious illness gives one a unique perspective on the world that is hard to describe to someone who has never been there. For the patient, the normal flow of life stops and the focus is now directed entirely on the self. Events seem to happen in slow motion and are usually permanently and vividly recorded in the memory. One often finds oneself looking at the outside world in amazement, marveling that it is going on about its business unaffected by the trauma of one's own life. One feels a sense of distance, of unreality, of being cut off from normal human intercourse, of apartness and separation. Serious illness is a shocking reminder that we are mortal and that our mortality involves an ultimate aloneness that is terrifying. I had often been touched when I taught the medieval play *Everyman* to my college sophomores by Everyman's reaction to the call from Death. After he had tried to bribe Death and realized he could not escape this time, he was beset with an overwhelming loneliness. If he had to go, he bargained with Death, at least could he take someone else with him? Only someone who has been seriously ill or who has been given a terminal diagnosis can understand that kind of existential loneliness and fear.

What one needs most in such times, as the anonymous author of *Everyman* well understood, is human companionship and love and support. I was somewhat comforted by the thought of my mother and father waiting for me downstairs, and I had been treated well in the outpatient department, but this present business was something else again. Most patients are heavily drugged before they go to surgery; consequently, they are pretty much oblivious to their surroundings and feel little anxiety. I was not drugged; consequently, I was totally aware of the assembly-line atmosphere that was all-pervasive. Everything I had experienced since going through those double doors into the surgical wing--the indifference of the attendants, lying in rows of stretchers, the waiting--all had converged to intensify the message that you had no significance as an individual, only as a disease, and that you were one of hundreds that had come in the past, that were presently there, and would come tomorrow.

I forced myself to look away from the windows and my morbid reflections, and to explore the rest of my surroundings. I could see that the operating rooms ran along the other side of the hall, each with its own scrub station in the hallway. I counted ten such set-ups that I could see from my horizontal position. Doctors walked by on their way to surgery discussing the techniques they would use, no one paying the slightest bit of attention to me or to the other patients similarly lined up in that hallway. Finally, a male nurse came over, and without even introducing himself, proceeded to shave the front left side of my head, right there in the hall. This time I was glad I was invisible to everyone else. I tried to shrink up into myself and pretend that this was not happening to me. I didn't even bother to try to deflect the embarrassment of the situation by talking to him. After he had finished, I was again left lying there for about three quarters of an hour before someone finally wheeled me into the operating room.

A young doctor followed me in, introduced himself as the assistant surgeon, called me *Doctor* Potts, which shocked me as medical doctors do not often bestow that title on mere Ph.D's, and proceeded to scrub the side of my shaved head with disinfectant for the next ten minutes. While he was working on my head, he began to discuss deconsruction (the latest theory in literary criticism), a conversation that struck me as thoroughly inappropriate, but at least it distracted me for a time. I was impressed that he had taken the time to read my chart carefully, to note my profession and my credentials and to talk to me about it. He was humane enough to acknowledge I had a life outside this room, indeed that I was a real person. He was one of the few people I met in Rochester who tried to cut through the impersonalization and to touch my uniqueness. I was immensely grateful. After he had finished sterilizing my head, the nurses proceeded to drape me, the surgeon I had met yesterday came in, and the operation began.

It was, as I had anticipated, unpleasant. Apart from the injection of the local anesthetic into the side of my head, it was not painful, but there is something distinctly unappetizing about having someone cutting open your head and using drills and laser cauterizers to cut out pieces of artery, when you are awake. They had promised me the surgery would only last about a half an hour, and they were right, although it seemed like three. At one point I could hear a whirling sound like a dentist's drill, and then I saw flashes of color from under my tent-like draping. The next thing I knew, sparks were dancing across my brain, and then someone began pulling and pushing deep inside my head. I gritted my teeth and tried to use some of my biofeedback relaxation techniques, but they really did not help. I was simply too tense.

I was so caught up in what they were doing to me that I forgot about the outcome. As they were sewing me up after what seemed an interminable amount of time, a piercing voice suddenly came over the microphone in the operating room and announced, "Potts, negative for arteritis." Apparently they had sent the sample of the artery to the lab and the technicians had already tested the tissue for disease. I blurted out from underneath the layers of draping, "Oh, no!", meaning we had gone through all this for nothing. Complete silence pervaded the operating room. With a thud, I realized they all thought I was disappointed that I did not have arteritis. I had been so confident of the diagnosis that I had not even considered a negative biopsy. Obviously, my reaction had taken everyone in that room aback, and it occurred to me that they all probably now thought I had made up the whole business. My sudden outburst conveyed the impression that I wanted to be sick, and the negative results had frustrated that desire.

I was mortified, but I was certainly in no position to explain or to justify myself. All I could do was keep quiet and tell myself that it would soon be over. Nobody said anything until the operation was finished. Asolute dead silence, except for the clicking of instruments and the occasional order from the surgeon. When they had finished sewing me up, and had bandaged my head and removed the draping, the surgeon's assistant took pity on me and tried to talk to me about the results.

"I know you very much need a diagnosis," he suggested, "but you really do not want to have arteritis. It is not nice."

He then told me he would call Dr. Campbell to tell him the results. A nurse rolled me back into the hall where I once again was left waiting. The assistant came back about ten minutes later and informed me that I had an appointment with Dr. Campbell back at the main Mayo Clinic building at two p.m. This assistant was young, and upon reflection, an obviously decent person. I am sorry now that I was too distraught and preoccupied to notice him further. He does, however, stand out in my memory, even though a shadowy figure on that terrible day, as a shining example of the humanity and compassion with which medical care can be dispensed.

I was soon wheeled back to outpatient recovery where Sister Sweeney and the recovery nurse were more than solicitous. They were both disappointed and concerned for me when I told them the doctors had found nothing and really tried to cheer me up. The nurse told me she always got upset when a patient came through her unit in chronic pain and the doctors could not find the cause. She helped me into one of the easy chairs, brought me a cup of coffee, and told me she wanted me to stay for an hour or so to make sure I was all right. She then called my father who was downstairs in the waiting room to tell him I would be down shortly.

That recovery room, apart from the bathroom outside 15W-B, was the friendliest place I had so far encountered in my stay in Rochester. The nurses who took care of us were super-nice, and the other patients who were recovering on either side of me--two young women who had had some kind of nerve surgery on their arms--were extra friendly as we chatted about the procedures we had just undergone. I seemed to be on some kind of unreal plateau during that short stay in outpatient recovery. I was relieved the procedure was over, and the consequences of the negative biopsy had not yet fully registered. I was actually beginning to enjoy myself until the anesthetic wore off. Then the pain slowly seeped into every nerve in my head. By the time I got dressed and a volunteer arrived to take me back downstairs in a wheelchair, I was really sick with the pain. Reality began to set in as I told my mother and father in the family waiting room that the biopsy was negative. They looked surprised, but said nothing.

We drove back to the motel in silence. I was too sick with the pain to offer any further explanations and I really did not want to talk about what had happened to me that morning. It had been too traumatic. I was busy trying to sort out my own emotions--humiliation, anger, frustration, confusion, embarrassment--and did not have enough left over to worry about those of my mother and father.

I got back to my room about eleven-thirty in the morning. I lay down on the bed and once again tried my biofeedback exercises as a way of relaxing down through the pain. But I was not very successful. I lay there quietly, trying not to think of anything, until just after one, the pain simmering. When I tried to stand up to get myself ready for my two p.m. appointment back at the clinic, I reeled from the renewed pain and a swirling dizziness engulfed me. It took a few minutes, standing and bracing myself against the dresser, for my head to clear. Finally, I looked at myself in the mirror. I didn't look as bad as I thought I would, but the very large dressing and bandage over the left side of my head was indeed unsightly. I thought about taking it off, then decided to be sensible. I gingerly placed the purple mesh scarf over the top of my head, fastened the ends behind my neck and surveyed the results. Not too bad, but still terribly conspicuous. I went next door to my parents' room, knocked on the door, and begged a ride back to the clinic.

The assistant surgeon had told me that morning to take aspirin if the pain got unbearable later in the day. I had taken two after I had returned to my motel room and two more just before I left for the clinic. As I settled in to the waiting room of 15W-B, I knew the aspirin were totally useless to combat what was going on inside my head. Taking aspirin to deal with that pain was like using a single bucket of water to douse a forest fire. Surely those surgeons knew that. As I sat there waiting, I reflected, seriously, for the first time, that doctors did not always know what they were doing, even at the Mayo Clinic. As two p.m. arrived, and then three, and then four, I was even more convinced. The pain was all-encompassing, almost beyond the point of endurance. I contemplated lying down on the floor, but my British sense of decorum would not allow it. I toyed with the idea of asking the nurses if there was somewhere I could lie down, but I was still too intimidated by the ambiance in that waiting room to ask for special favors. For all my education and teaching experience, I am still not an assertive person, especially in a situation where I am the supplicant. Those nurses were far too efficient and impersonal to be approached for special privileges. Instead, I focused my entire energies on lasting five more minutes, and then five more, and then five more, praying I would not disgrace myself by fainting. I should have picked up the signal that I was no longer a priority for anybody at this clinic, but I didn't.

It was not until five p.m. that I was finally ushered in to see Dr. Campbell. He charged into his office/examining room and sat down at his desk, appearing distracted and busy. After a minute or two of shuffling papers, he turned his attention to me, looked at my bandaged head and asked me if I were in pain. I looked back at him in shock, then hung my head. I could barely reply, stunned at the absolute stupidity of the question.

Then Dr. Campbell became business-like as he toyed with my records on his desk, and told me I should go home and try a pain-management center. He did not look at me; instead, he busied himself with writing notations on my records. I did not catch on immediately that I was being dismissed, so I started to ask him questions about possible illnesses other than arteritis. He was evasive and would not answer me directly. He still did not look at me. Whenever I asked him a direct question, he replied by asking me for my internist's address at home and said he would write a report to him. After this interchange had occurred three times, I finally realized he was not going to pursue my case any further and wanted to be rid of me. With horror, I demanded to know if he was suggesting my illness was psychosomatic. He merely shrugged his shoulders and became cold and distant. Feebly, I repeated some of my complaints, like "I have headaches," and, "my neck hurts," which finally tumbled off into monosyllables as I understood the futility of any further appeals. He did look at me once, finally, and suggested that since giant cell arteritis tends to jump around, they could biopsy the other side of my head. I mumbled something about that side not hurting, although at the moment, my whole head hurt and was swimming in a dizzying, stinging circle.

At one point in our verbal sparring, Dr. Campbell looked out the window and mused for a moment, telling me they had discovered the same abnormal protein readings that had registered at home. But then I could visibly see him chucking aside that particular lab result, probably because he didn't know what to do with it, and he had decided he was finished with me. I had already taken up too much of his time. He mumbled something about unresolved personal problems in my life, then he suggested that the left temporal headaches could have come from grinding my teeth. I jumped and exclaimed that I did not grind my teeth, but he waved me to silence. Then, as a final blow, he intimated that my problems could come from drinking too much. He told me the rheumatologist had suggested this interesting possibility based on a mild macrositis (enlarged red blood cells) which had shown up on one of the blood tests. And I did admit that I had abused alcohol on the MMPI, didn't I? That test was lurking in the background, giving me a sick nauseating feeling in the pit of my stomach.

This last insult undid me. I had been humiliated enough for one day, and now to be charged with alcoholism was beyond enduring. Yes, I drink, I told him, but not excessively. The suggestion that alcohol was the source of my problems was simply not true, I insisted. He sat there, nodding smugly. I finally just sat there too, looking at him in stunned silence and impotent humiliation. All active alcoholics insist they are not alcoholics, and I knew that the more loudly and vehemently I protested my innocence, the more I would underscore my guilt.

He was maddeningly in control and there was nothing I could do about it. Whenever I attempted to regain any kind of composure during this last interview by suggesting further evaluations, or other possibilities, Dr. Campbell put me off by repeating his promise to write a report to my internist at home, and that I should follow up with him. We ended my Mayo Clinic experience when he finally became solicitous of my pain and offered to get me three Darvocet pills to get me through until the next morning. Addictive personalities obviously cannot handle narcotic drugs, I thought bitterly. Collecting whatever dignity I could muster, I stumbled out of his office, picked up my cashier's receipt at the front desk and fled the Mayo Clinic. It had never occurred to me, never in a thousand years, that this would happen. Stung with humiliation, I now had to face my mother and father and tell them I was a fake. I would now have to admit to them that all their worry and anxiety over me was groundless, and that I was a whining, hopeless neurotic and an alcoholic. Even though I had a fleeting instinct that none of these things were true, I was beyond common sense at that point in time as I was overcome with a groundwash of humiliation and paranoia.

CHAPTER SEVEN

LATE JUNE, 1985

It was now Friday, June 21, 1985. I had first become ill in July, 1984, almost a year ago, and from my perspective, it appeared that the medical profession had given up on me. As far as I was concerned, they had thrown up their hands in despair, had placed the blame firmly back on me, and then had closed ranks. As Dr. Campbell went over my case with me during that last interview at the Mayo Clinic, I watched him take each one of my symptoms in turn, disassociate it from any kind of pattern and trivialize it. The left temporal headaches were probably caused by grinding my teeth, the enlarged red blood cells were from drinking too much, and the elevated sed rate was probably normal for me. He described it as being only "slightly" elevated. I noted the adjective well, an obvious attempt at minimizing this specific piece of evidence. He likewise dismissed the abnormal protein electrophoresis results as too general to say anything and suggested that test was probably a red herring. Finally, the neck pain and headaches were little more than tension caused by unresolved problems in my personal life. What he did not tell me was that I also had a positive antinuclear antibody blood test and a low white blood cell count, both significant findings in a diagnosis of collagen diseases and two of the diagnostic criteria for systemic lupus. By themselves, neither test said much because they were borderline abnormal, but together, and added to the elevated sed rate and the abnormal protein electrophoresis, they were clear warnings of an autoimmune disease. This diagnosis should have been even more obvious in the light of my medical history and the symptoms I had described, but since the latter could not be quantified in lab tests, Dr. Campbell apparently discounted them.

To this day, I honestly do not know why he dismissed me as neurotic; probably a combination of the MMPI results and the rheumatologist's assessment of my symptoms as functional, although this conclusion is sheer speculation on my part. Nor was there any doubt as to his convictions. His brusque attitude clearly conveyed to me the impression that I had wasted his time, and had somehow manipulated him into thinking my case was urgent. His annoyance with me was obvious during that last interview. He would not look at me, nor give me any kind of reassurance, on any level. And his summation of the test results was cursory, to say the least. He told me about the sed rate and blood protein, and then said that since the EMG (muscle conduction test) was negative, there was no need for a muscle biopsy. Any further results he would include in his report; he did not want to discuss them further with me at that moment. He clearly indicated he had no more time to give me and was no longer interested in my physical distress. Nor did he suggest any future treatment or symptoms to watch for, implying that such action was unnecessary. Try as I might, there was nothing I could say or do to reassert my credibility. Nor did I even have the luxury of being angry, as he had been doing me a favor by taking me on as an extra patient. Mayo Clinic doctors are on salary, so it was not to his advantage to continue testing. We parted in dead silence.

Ramada Inns had recently been running an ad on television emphasizing the superior quality of their service. A poor, exhausted client checked in to the competition's motel, dragged his three heavy suitcases down hall after hall, finally found what he thought was his room, panting and sweating, only to go through the door and find himself back out in the parking lot in front of a hamper of dirty linens. The analogy to my exhausting search struck me as apt. Many times I had struggled down those same dark corridors, trying various doors, and had finally found the one that seemed to open up to some answers about my illness. The relief as I went through the door was immense, but three times, already, I had found myself back out in that parking lot.

After I left Dr. Campbell's office and had picked up my cashier's receipt, I blindly made my way to the bank of telephones down the hall to call my mother to come and get me. When I tried to tell her what happened, I started choking and knew I was on the edge of losing control. She told me my father had already driven to the clinic to get me, and I was to wait there for him. I could hear her voice growing distant, which always happens when she doesn't know what to make of a situation. I hung up and found my father further down the hall. I can always control myself in front of him, so I told him, as clinically as I could, that the clinic doctors felt there was nothing wrong with me. He accepted my superficial and edited explanation, and seemed to be relieved. We chatted trivia on the way back to the motel, making plans to leave in the morning for Canada.

Once back in my motel room and finally alone, I thought I would break down, but I didn't. I sat in a chair for awhile, and then ran a tub full of hot water, lay in it, and soaked. I was amazed at my control. I felt a dull, heavy, emotional aching in my chest, and of course the usual physical pain, but no releasing tears. After I got out of the tub, I put on my nightgown and housecoat and went next door to tell my mother and father to go to dinner without me. I was far too upset to eat. I think they were relieved as they did not know what to say or how to deal with me. Then I sat down to write an account to Dale of what had happened to me. He had made me promise I would call him if "they" started giving me a hard time in Rochester, an interesting premonition. He was the only person I had talked to extensively about my illness, and I now had a desperate need to communicate with him. The letter would also give him a couple of weeks to think about the situation before I saw him again.

After I had finished the letter, I put on my slippers and went down to the lobby to mail it. Patients wandered all over the halls in their housecoats. Rochester is not your typical tourist town. As I walked through the front lobby, I passed a cigarette machine and stopped. I stood there looking at it for a good two minutes and probably would have bought some if I had had any money on me. The urge had passed by the time I got back to my room, however, no thanks to my self-discipline. Then the phone started to ring. The first call was from Sister Sweeney. She was really concerned abut the negative results of the biopsy, had called to see if I was okay, and was shocked when I told her I had been dismissed. I thanked her for her concern and hung up, as close to tears as I could come. But again I did not cry. Nor was I to do so for a very long time.

The Mayo Clinic verdict had put an authoritative stamp on my non-illness that was to effectively deny me any of the legitimate emotional expressions that accompany illness for many months to come. I could not feel unhappy, nor depressed, nor angry, nor could I cry, because I was not ill. The Mayo Clinic had said so. Whenever I would find myself on the edge of tears, I would jolt back, remembering I was not allowed. This reaction was not a conscious choice; it was a conditioned response brought on by the Mayo Clinic's *ex cathedra* pronouncement. An interesting article by Timothy Anderson and David Helm describes the physician-patient encounter as a process of reality negotiation, in which medical practitioners and institutions create a social reality of what is "health" and what is "illness," often distinct from any physical reality. The patient brings his or her symptoms to the doctor and argues for the sick role, which the doctor then allows or disallows. Within this illness role, certain behaviors are appropriate, such as grief, irritability, the giving up of responsibilities at school, at work and as a family member. Such behaviors are not condoned, however, if one has not been sanctioned as ill by Medicine.[1] Hence, I could not cry. It would take months of Dale's gentle counselling and a violent emotional upheaval to convince me that I had a right to be sick, in spite of what the Mayo Clinic had said. And even then, I could not cry.

Then, one of my colleagues who was also a friend called from home, and when I told her what had happened, that I was told there was nothing wrong with me, she flew into a rage, a "hissy fit" as she refers to them. She called the Mayo Clinic every four letter word in her vocabulary, which was extensive, and when she ran out, she started again. Had I not been in semi-shock, I would have been amused. When her anger finally sputtered out, she told me to take care of myself and I hung up. Then Irene called. Her reaction was silence. After that, I stopped answering the phone. I was simply not up to telling anybody else from home what the Mayo Clinic doctors had said. Let them tell each other, I thought. My mother and father appeared at my door about nine p.m. with some soup, a hot roll and some tea on a tray, but I couldn't eat anything. The food simply wouldn't go past the aching in my throat. Instead, I drank the tea, took one of my precious Darvocet pills, and went to bed. I fell into an exhausted sleep almost immediately.

I woke up the next morning feeling better for the rest and surveyed myself in the mirror. That bandage looked terrible, so I took it off. The wound was about three and a half inches long, from just above the middle of my left ear up the side of my head and across the temple. With proper styling, I could pull the hair on the left side forward enough to cover the damage, but I needed to wash it. It was caked with blood and gel and antiseptic all around the shaved area and was sticking straight out. The assistant surgeon had told me the stitches

[1]Timothy Anderson and David Helm, "The Physician-Patient Encounter: A Process of Reality Negotiation" in Jaco, *Patients, Physicians, and Illness*, 261 ff.

would dissolve on their own in a few days, but I had to be careful of infection in the meantime. Hence I was not to get the area wet. Finally, I hit on an idea. I filled the tub full of water, got in it, and lay down on my right side. I put a small towel over the wound and then lowered the right side of my head into the water as far as I dared. It was awkward, but I managed to clean the caked areas without getting the wound wet and to wash the rest of my hair. Then I got out of the tub, dressed, toweled my hair dry, and arranged it to cover the stitches as best as I could. I didn't even need one of the scarves. The damage would be almost unnoticeable, as long as I stayed out of the wind.

Dealing with this practical necessity distracted me for a time from the next order of business. I had to make one more trip back to the clinic in order to settle my account before we left Rochester, and I was not looking forward to it. It was an effort to make myself go back into that building, but I did it. I had to wait for an hour before one of the twenty-odd uniformed cashiers was free, and as I sat there in the large waiting area of the lobby adjacent to the cashier's area, I watched all the patients coming and going with mixed feelings. Many would certainly be helped by the Mayo Clinic doctors, but I wondered how many would be peremptorily dismissed as I had been, thrown back on their own resources to deal with the terrible emotional repercussions of having been labelled neurotic, as well as having to continue the search elsewhere for a cause for their illness. Some, I knew, would probably give up. Once again I had cause to meditate on the immense power the medical profession has over our lives. As Anderson and Helm point out, the individual patient is the one who knows himself better than anyone else, but in a medical encounter, the physician has the power to illegitimize the patient's condition and to discredit him.[2] I was leaving Rochester in a worse state than when I had arrived because on top of my physical problems, I now had to deal with having been discredited by one of the most prestigious medical institutions in our country.

We left town immediately and began the drive up to Canada to my family's summer home in the Muskoka Lakes north of Toronto. Exhausted from the surgery and emotional strain, I lay in the back seat of the car and slept for the entire two-day drive. I slept partly as an escape from having to deal with the verdict, and partly from the effects of the Darvocet and the whole exhausting experience. Once we got into Canada, I replenished my supply of narcotics with "222's," a mixture of aspirin and codeine that is available over the counter in Canada. I needed the drug to maintain the emotional stupor I had achieved as much as to dull the physical pain. The codeine, interestingly enough, emptied my mind, and as long as I was emotionally blank, I could not feel the awesome rejection I had just suffered. I took far more than I should have, but I really did not care about being sensible. All I cared about was not hurting, emotionally or physically. I was not yet ready to face the future and to start thinking about what to do next.

We arrived at our summer home late Friday evening, and I spent the next two weeks sitting by the lake meditating. My family all walked on tiptoe, carefully avoiding any discussion of the situation in front of me. I trusted no one and would confide in no one. I was afraid if I started discussing the experience

[2]Anderson and Helm, *"The Physician-Patient Encounter, 269.*

we would all have to admit up front that I had wasted everybody's emotional energy. I was not about to articulate that possibility, thereby endorsing what I knew they all thought but were afraid to say. I was, irrationally, angry with every one of them, I suppose because they were convenient. I was angry with them for not being indignant on my behalf, for not openly supporting me, and for not helping me search out solutions. I now know they were as confused as I was, and my surly withdrawal made them cautious. They did talk about it, however, when they thought I was asleep. One evening I overheard my mother warning my brothers and sister that I would not tolerate any hint of a suggestion that my problems were emotional, not physical. "Damn right," I said to myself, "and just let any one of you try it!" The only time I dared acknowledge my physical condition occurred one day as I was ironing in the living room. The pain in the muscles down the back of my neck and down my shoulders was particularly acute, thudding and throbbing. I remarked to my mother that if I had made all this up, I sure had a powerful imagination. She just sighed.

Halfway through my visit, we drove up to the north side of Lake Superior for a family reunion in a small mining town called Wawa (Indian for wild goose). Many of my relatives lived in this northern area of Ontario, and, while I usually enjoyed their company, I was in no mood for festivities. They all carefully circled around my problems, except for one cousin who, after observing me for a couple of days, took me aside and said, "Are you sure they didn't find anything wrong? You are obviously in pain and you look sick." I could have kissed him. But he was the only one who openly endorsed my condition.

I did not fully recognize how strung out I was emotionally until the first night of the reunion. I was staying in a motel that was built in log-cabin style, picturesque, but certainly not sound proof. The logs separating the rooms were solid enough, but the mortar between them was paper thin. Four young men had come in from the bush to celebrate Canada Day (July 1). They were determined to have a good time and partied all night, in spite of the fact that partying had been expressly forbidden by the management. The television and stereo blared most of the night, and every time one of them went in or out, that door slammed like a thunderclap. I called the front desk some four times in the course of the night and finally around six a.m., close to hysterics, I called again and asked the desk clerk who was going to call the police, her or me? She did. I also called over to an adjacent separate cabin where my mother and father were staying with my brother and his family and pleaded for help. My brother, all 210 pounds of him and dressed in nothing but a raggedy old pair of jeans, ambled sleepily across the dirt roadway to my room, listened to the noise, and knocked on their door. When one of them opened it, he demanded, "Are you guys assholes by nature, or do you practice?" I warned him there were four of them, and that he had better cool it. Just then, the police arrived, thank God, and hauled them all away by the ears. Before they left, however, the police made them apologize to me. They did, and appeared sincerely repentant.

Under normal circumstances, I would have readily forgiven the truants, as I could see they were good kids and were just blowing off steam. And I probably would have found my brother's bravado and colorful language amusing, as it now appears to me. But I was not capable of responding sensibly or with good nature. I started shaking uncontrollably, which frightened everybody, including me. I went across the roadway to the other cabin, had some tea and

English muffins with my mother, and took two Xanax (tranquilizers), trying to calm down. It took about a half hour before I could feel the drug working, and then went back to my room and slept all morning. I did wonders for the festive spirit of that family reunion.

The final day of the get-together, we all drove to my cousin's summer cottage on the shores of Lake Superior for a barbecue and fishing expedition. The scenery was post-card perfect: crystal clear water, a robin's egg-blue sky, and the deep green of the northern Canadian forest. It was one of those precious days that Canadians cherish, when the weather is soft and warm and caressing, the days that one remembers when it is fifteen degrees below zero and one is huddled against the cruelties of the far-northern climate. My father and brother talked me into going fishing with them, so we commandeered my cousin's battered aluminum boat, powered by a beat-up fifteen-h.p.-Evinrude outboard motor, and began quietly to troll about a half-mile offshore. We didn't say anything to each other, each one of us lost in the utter beauty and serenity of the landscape, and our own thoughts. I was struck by the incongruity of my emotional inner turmoil with the peaceful external world and silently prayed to whatever God had made all this beauty to please help me. A few minutes later, my line bobbed and I was thunderstruck as I realized I had actually hooked a fish. I hadn't thought it through that far, that when you go fishing you might catch something. I was too stupid to do anything about the situation, so my brother took my line and brought the fish in--a nice two-pound, fresh-water salmon. I was thrilled, and for a moment forgot my troubles. Then, as we were heading for shore, I prayed once again that maybe the fish was a good omen, that perhaps there was an answer somewhere down the road if I could just persevere.

Back at our summer home a few days later, however, rather than confronting the rest of my family with my problems which would have been the healthy thing to do, I again took refuge in silence. Ruth and Larry called one day, to see what had happened in Rochester. They were in Toronto visiting relatives and were anxious to know what the Mayo Clinic doctors had found. When I told them what had happened, they were confused and did not know how to respond to me. Larry kept repeating, "They found nothing?" I also talked to Stephen, and when I told him the Mayo Clinic doctors could find nothing wrong with me, he innocently replied, "That's good, huh?"

CHAPTER EIGHT

JULY, 1985--SEPTEMBER, 1985

I flew back to Texas two weeks later, still nursing my self-destructive bitterness, but determined that I was not beaten. As I kissed my father goodbye at the airport, he cheerfully announced that now I could go home and put all the bad times behind me. I was cured. I was not particularly hurt that he had bought the Mayo Clinic verdict because I knew he didn't want me to be ill. It would be hard for anybody to reject the assessment of an institution such as the Mayo Clinic, let alone a worried parent. But I could not accept their conclusions. After carefully examining my bruised body and soul, I had decided I had been sold a bill of goods. The physical evidence of my symptoms was too real and too persistent to dismiss as nervous tension. Something was physically wrong with my body, I did not do it to myself, and somewhere out there was a doctor who would find it. Larry, God bless him, had kept telling me it would take the right person at the right time, and I clung to that hope.

On the way home in the plane, I decided I would keep an appointment I had made with Dr. Madrid, the neurologist who had examined me the previous summer in the hospital when I had first become ill. I had made the appointment at Dale's urging in early May when it appeared Dr. Silverman's needles would never arrive and that we were at a standstill. Dale worked closely with Dr. Madrid and had a great deal of confidence in him. I had also been impressed when I read the report he had written. His was the only one in my medical records that was accurate, complete, well-written, and insightful. When I had called in May, Dr. Madrid's secretary had told me I could not get an appointment until July 11. I went ahead and made the appointment, not really thinking I would need it, sure I would come up with some answers long before then. In the haste to get to Rochester and the subsequent emotional reaction to the way they had treated me, I had forgotten about Dr. Madrid. Now, he seemed like my only hope. I had to do something, I told a friend who picked me up at the airport. I still felt sick, and as long as the symptoms persisted, I would go on searching. Part of it was stubbornness, but a much larger motivation was fear. Something was terribly awry with my body, not like the ordinary sicknesses such as the 'flu, even pneumonia, that I had experienced before. This was different, and I was terrified that whatever it was that was eating away at my insides would get serious before I could get someone's attention.

When I got home, I called Bill Collins and conveyed to him my disappointment at the Mayo Clinic experience. "Don't feel that way," he reassured me. It is not any of those awful diseases we thought you had."

"What is it then?" I asked him.

"Muscles. Tension," he replied.

I felt a sinking feeling in the pit of my stomach. He was on their side. He didn't believe me either.

Then he told me he wanted me to start on a new drug, an amitriptyline tricyclic called Elavil that would help the pain. I copied down the name of the drug, making a mental note to look it up in the *Physicians' Desk Reference* later that afternoon, and told him I wanted to do one more thing before I let them lock me up in a psychiatric ward. I wanted to see Dr. Madrid. Bill readily agreed, he had no objections, but when I asked him to send on a copy of the Mayo Clinic report he had just received to Dr. Madrid, he refused outright. He told me he would talk to him about it, but he would not give it to him.

Startled and suspicious, I hung up the phone and sat at my dining room table for a good ten minutes before I could get up. Why was he being so uncooperative and secretive about that report? And why had he not suggested I drop by so that we could talk about my problems? Dr. Campbell at the Mayo Clinic must have done quite a number on me, I speculated. Giving Bill the benefit of the doubt, I decided he was only trying to protect me. But now I really felt frustrated. Dr. Campbell would not talk to me in any depth about all the tests that they had run, deferring that job to my own internist. And here he was refusing to do it either. Apparently, Bill Collins' pronouncement that my problem was tension was all I was going to get. That afternoon I went to the library, got out the *PDR* and looked up Elavil. There it was. An antidepressant. Not only that, it was exactly the same drug I had been on since January (Endep), only a different brand name. Once again, my stomach sunk down to my ankles. I had had a great number of bad experiences with doctors in the year that I had been ill, but I had never felt betrayed the way I did sitting there that day in the reference room of the library, staring at the Elavil entry in the *PDR*.

That same afternoon, I went to see Dale. I was nervous about going because I did not know what kind of reception awaited me. If he tried to reconcile me to the Mayo Clinic verdict, I knew I would bottom out. I should have been more trustful. I was barely seated in his recliner chair when he started apologizing for the Mayo Clinic in particular and for the entire medical profession in general. "I know it must have been a demoralizing, totally humiliating experience for you," he said, and started apologizing all over again. When I pointed out that it was difficult to discount what an institution such as the Mayo Clinic had said, he turned on me. "They have done a pretty good character assassination on you," he almost shouted. "Don't do it to yourself as well!" He told me he and Dr. Madrid had gone over the copy of the notebook I had left behind, and that they had both been totally confident I would come back with a diagnosis. Dr. Madrid had agreed he would take over my case and treat whatever it was the Mayo Clinic had found. Dale said he had been stunned when he got my letter and his first reaction was concern for me. He was afraid I would blow my brains out. I was touched by his concern, and assured him I was not suicidal, yet.

Then Dale told me that after he had received my letter, he had reviewed my notebook, his notes from all our sessions together, and had thought much about my case. He had decided my illness was not psychosomatic, that I had a genuine physical problem and that we needed to go on looking. He explained that the research literature suggested most patients diagnosed as psychosomatic develop quantifiable evidence of disease within two years, and that doctors are far too ready to use the label psychosomatic when they are stumped. "However, I have been wrong before," he warned me, "although I do not think I am wrong this time." He told me I must, absolutely must, keep the appointment with Dr. Madrid, and that he would telephone him first and warn him about what had happened. He told me he would suggest to Dr. Madrid that he clear his appointments before and after mine so that I would not be rushed, and so that he could spend time with me. Dale's total trust in me did marvels for my self-assurance, and I felt much better after I left him. But I was not looking forward to the interview with Dr. Madrid.

Two days later, July 11, I kept my appointment with Dr. Madrid. He was doctor number sixteen I had consulted, and by this time, although hopeful, I was suspicious and wary. My appointment was in the office he used on Wednesday afternoons, on the west side of town near the university. After I had driven there, I sat in my car in the parking lot for a full five minutes before I could bring myself to get out of the car and go in the building. He was in the secretaries' section, behind the glass that separates patients from office workers, and as soon as I saw him, I turned on my heels, left the office and went back to my car. I sat there again for another five minutes, telling myself that I was being childish, and, mustering a supreme effort, I finally went back in. Thank God he was no longer behind that glass. I told the secretary who I was, and almost immediately, Dr. Madrid appeared at the door to the inner office. He took me to his personal office immediately, himself, which impressed me. Most doctors do not descend to this level. They wait in their offices for you to be led to them by a clerk/servant. Somewhat slimmed down and more subdued than the last time I had met him, he sat and listened to my nervous recital, reviewed the medical history and lab reports Dale had given him, examined me, and said yes, something was wrong. He told me this was not the first time he had disagreed with the Mayo Clinic, but he needed a copy of the report, of their findings. I had to admit that Bill Collins would not release it, and that we would have to approach the Mayo Clinic directly. He seemed put off that we had to go to that trouble, but insisted he needed it immediately. I signed a release form and he suggested a muscle biopsy as the next step. Apparently, we were still considering a muscle disease. Reluctantly, I agreed. He put me back on Prednisone, the same drug Dr. Silverman had used, and told me to call him if I experienced any side effects.

After I had left Dr. Madrid's office, I was considerably cheered. Thanks to Dale, he had reacted with the appropriate indignation at the Mayo Clinic's handling of my case and seemed genuinely interested in pursuing the matter. With infinite relief, I realized he believed me, and I felt he would be aggressive in pursuing answers. I did not particularly want to go through another invasive medical procedure, but I had to trust him. The number of people who still had faith in me was diminishing. My family was ambivalent, I knew where Collins stood, and many of my friends had made it clear upon my return that they had bought into the Mayo Clinic myth. Some even openly told me it was time I acted like an adult and accepted the psychosomatic origins to my complaints. I had Dale, Larry, and Ruth, and one or two other friends who were loyal. And now Dr. Madrid. I had the biopsy a week later on my right upper arm.

I decided I did not want to have the surgery at the hospital I usually dealt with because I knew too many people there, and I did not want to run into Bill Collins. He had strongly advised against the biopsy, insisting it was unnecessary. We arranged for me to go through another hospital on the other side of town, once again as an outpatient. Dr. Madrid warned me it would hurt as they could only give me a superficial local anesthetic. I did not like that idea at all and thought about it a great deal while I was waiting. You never get used to pain, so I discovered. In addition to the anticipated pain, I was also apprehensive about another surgical routine and the accompanying humiliations as I subjected myself to clerks and nurses and unfamiliar doctors, so soon after the terrible experience in Rochester. Nor was I particularly hopeful that they would find anything. I had had so many negative test results, I held out little hope for this one. I could not, however, afford to alienate Dr. Madrid by refusing the biopsy. I had to do some serious work on my attitude to make myself show up on the appointed day.

When Ruth offered to drive me to the hospital, I quickly accepted. I did not think I would be in any condition to drive myself home, and besides, I needed the moral support. She picked me up at my house at six-thirty a.m., and we got to the hospital around seven. Just before she dropped me off, she told me Larry said not to worry about the pain. There were few nerve endings inside muscle, and I probably would feel little discomfort. I thanked her, got out of the car, and headed for the front door of the hospital and all I knew was waiting for me inside.

A young technician, half my age, took my insurance information at the main outpatient office, and then proceeded to draw blood and weigh me. She then handed me a plastic cup and told me she needed a urine sample. I had visited the ladies' room before checking in to the office, so I told her she would have to wait on that one. She shrugged, told me not to bother, and threw the cup away. Chalk one up for our side, I thought. At least I won't have to pay for that one unnecessary test. Then a teenaged volunteer led me upstairs to surgery. Yesterday, or any other day, the hospital staff would assume I was adult enough to find it on my own, as Ruth was to do three hours later when she returned to get me. But not today; not as a patient. I could feel myself starting to get irritated already and had to use some self-discipline not to take it out on the candy-striper.

Once I got into the outpatient waiting area, I discovered that the process was much more intimate than what I had experienced in Rochester. Once again depositing my clothes in a locker and putting on a hospital gown, cap, and slippers, I walked over to the nearest stretcher and got on. There were only eight of them lined up along the wall. And there was only one other patient besides myself. The nurses, who were far more personable than those in the surgical waiting area at the hospital in Rochester, hitched up the back of the stretcher and brought me a magazine and coffee while I was waiting. About a half-hour later, the surgeon came in, cheerfully poked my right arm a few times until we found a muscle that hurt, and then directed the nurses to wheel me in to an operating room across the hall. I now knew the routine backwards. They draped me, bathed my upper arm in disinfectant, injected a local anesthetic into the right bicep, which hurt, and proceeded to cut into the muscle. Larry was right. I felt little pain, and the unpleasantness nowhere approached the biopsy on my head. The procedure lasted less than a half hour and I was soon back in outpatient recovery drinking coffee again. I still felt no pain, even after the anesthetic had worn off. Ruth came back for me about ten-thirty, helped me dress, and drove me home.

The whole procedure had little effect on me physically or emotionally, until I got the bill. Then I had apoplexy. The total, not counting the surgeon's fee, was exactly triple what the Mayo Clinic had charged me for a much more complex procedure. At least the Mayo Clinic is cost effective. I have since learned to estimate my medical expenses by calculating a horrendous amount, and then tripling it. I took the bill to the surgeon who went over it carefully with me, and he agreed that I had been taken. Every item on the bill was grossly inflated, and some were listed twice. I had no idea if they had indeed used all these supplies. One I was sure of, however. They listed a dressing for ten dollars (really a bandaid), which I knew they had not used. And they charged me something like five hundred per cent above the normal price. Obviously, they had padded my bill because I had insurance.

I called the business office of the hospital many times. They said they would have their auditors check the bill and would call me back, but they never did. Even if they did, I was sure they would find nothing out of line. Using their own auditors is a bit like sending the wolf in to guard the sheep pen I thought to myself. I even called my insurance company to find out what they considered a reasonable amount for such a procedure in my area, but they told me they did not give out such information to patients. When I argued I was trying to save them some money, that I needed the information if I was to argue persuasively about the exorbitant bill, the clerk just repeated that it was not their policy to give out such information to patients. So I gave up. In the end, they paid the bill in full, fools that they were, and I let the matter drop.

Then I settled in to wait for the results of the biopsy. A week passed and I called Dr. Madrid's secretary. No, the results had not yet come in. She would call me when they did. I waited another week; still no answer. A third week passed, and then a fourth. At last, at the end of the fifth week, the secretary decided to investigate and found that the results had been sent to the surgeon's office and got buried under a mound of paper work. She was sorry, and would have Dr. Madrid call me that afternoon. He did, told me the biopsy was negative, and to come by and see him to discuss where to go from there. I made an appointment to see him a week later.

It was now September, and a new school semester had started. The depression and fatigue that had plagued me from the beginning had intensified. And the depression increased as I waited week after week for the biopsy results. I began to suspect that Dr. Madrid's initial enthusiasm had waned. My appointment was in his east-side office, which was a zoo. His specialty was child neurology, so he kept a toy box for the children in one corner of his tiny waiting room. This particular day he was running way behind schedule, and when I arrived, the office was full of people, some of whom had been waiting two hours and more. The children were fighting over the toys, with each other, and kept running between the lobby of the building and the waiting room. Their screaming when they were disciplined did wonders for my headaches.

When I was finally ushered into Dr. Madrid's office by a most harried secretary, after an hour and a half wait, he handed me a copy of the biopsy report. It did not say much, only that the muscle tissue was normal. When I queried him about his reaction to the Mayo Clinic assessment, he looked startled. Apparently, he had never sent away for it, despite the urgency he had expressed five weeks previously. Obviously, he had forgotten about it as soon as I had disappeared. I signed another release form and tried to be philosophical. After all, how many students had spilled out their guts in my office, relating to me terribly personal things, and I had forgotten about them by the time I had arrived home that evening. Once again I was confronted with a basic fact of life when dealing with the medical profession. What was a crisis for me was routine for Dr.Madrid, and there was no reason to think I should have a special hold on this doctor's attention.

About a week before I had gone to see Dr. Madrid, a graduate student of mine who had heard of my problems had come to my office one day to share some of her similar experiences before she was diagnosed as having rheumatoid arthritis. She gave me a book to read that constituted another landmark in my search, *Understanding Arthritis*, put out by the American Arthritis Foundation. I literally devoured the book, especially the opening chapters that carefully explained the workings of the immune system and autoimmune diseases. The various chapters on different rheumatic diseases were short and obviously intended for the lay person, but they were a valuable first step for me. The text covered sixteen different forms of arthritis, and as I read through them, I stumbled across systemic lupus for the first time. I was interested in the description of this disease, as I was in all of them, but I did not seriously entertain it as a possibility. As I read through the book, I discovered that many rheumatic disorders are protean in their manifestations, are impossibly difficult to diagnose, and ornery to treat. I also found out that having a negative test result did not meant you made up a symptom, only that it eliminated a specific alternative. While this may seem like a simplistic notion to any physician, it was a revolutionary idea to me.

So, when Dr. Madrid told me the muscle biopsy was negative, I was prepared. It meant I did not have polymyositis or dermatomyositis, but I could still have polymyalgia rheumatica, despite what the Mayo Clinic doctors had said, because in that condition, all the tests usually came back negative. The only problem with that diagnosis was that I was too young. You had to be over sixty to get that one. I convinced myself that I did indeed have polymyalgia rheumatica because I desperately needed a label, but when I presented my diagnosis to Dr. Madrid that day he would not buy it. Instead, he suggested I fly to St. Louis to see the man who wrote the definitive book on muscle diseases. I was shocked. Another doctor, and another biopsy? And in St. Louis? After the Mayo Clinic experience, I was not about to subject myself to another "expert," so I tried to deflect this suggestion. He did, however, talk me into seeing yet another local doctor, this time a rheumatologist, a Dr. Gerald Wagner. I went home and mechanically made the appointment for September 16. When the day came, I can remember dragging myself to his office like an unwilling schoolgirl. I went, simply because I did not know what else to do.

I did not like Dr. Wagner's waiting room. It was terribly small, and he had the chairs in three rows, the first one against the wall and the second one facing it. There was not enough room between these two rows for patients to sit facing each other unless they interlocked their knees. Anybody who had tried to sit out there would have discovered the problem immediately. Neither Dr. Wagner nor his partner had apparently ever tried. I hoped this arrangement was not a premonition of things to come.

I was by now thoroughly conditioned to the routine in doctors' offices, so when Dr. Wagner's nurse called me out of the waiting room and escorted me to the scales, weighed me, led me to an examination room and told me to take off my clothes and to put on a paper nightie, I did so with a dull obedience. Then she took my pulse and blood pressure and asked me what drugs I was on. She made a note of my answer on a blank sheet of paper with my name typed on top, the beginnings of yet another set of medical records in yet another doctor's office. As she left, she told me the doctor would come in shortly. I sat on the side of the examining table and surveyed the room, almost identical to the countless others I had been in over the past year. On one side of the room sat the inevitable examining table with its paper runner, on another were side tables on which were arranged jars of cotton balls, tongue depressors and other miscellaneous medical paraphernalia, and on the third wall, a sink, and a couple of hard-backed, kitchen-type chairs. This particular room announced Dr. Wagner's specialty with wall posters put out by drug companies of swollen joints, a plaster model of a skeletal hand and foot on one of the tables, together with a cardboard chart on which were mounted samples of the various anti-inflammatory drugs available on the market.

After I had waited about ten minutes, Dr. Wagner appeared on the scene. He was reserved, professional and most business-like as he introduced himself and asked what he could do for me. Then, he sat down on one of the hard-backed chairs, looked at me expectantly, and I launched into my recital with little feeling. I expected nothing of him, and as I wearily recounted the details of the past year, I suppose I conveyed my mistrust. He took copious notes, asked me pointed questions here and there, and then examined me, as I had expected he would. When he remarked that I seemed most familiar with medical terminology and knew a great deal about medicine, I pointed out that I had had a year's schooling. He did all the usual things like listening to my heart and lungs, looking in my eyes, ears, nose, testing my reflexes, probing at my belly; but there were some new ones. He manipulated each one of my joints, especially those in my fingers and wrists and shoulders and feet. To my surprise, some of my finger joints hurt, but not much. He also asked me if I had ever had a rash-like reaction to the sun, and I innocently replied yes. I always broke out in a hive-like rash whenever I sat out in the sun, but I had never thought anything about it. Dr. Wagner made no comment. He finished his examination, and in spite of my world-weariness, I still had enough spark left to be bemused by the dynamics of the situation. Here I was, talking about a long-standing, searing, intensely-personal experience to a man I had never met before in my life, and I had nothing on except a paper nightie. He sure had all the advantages. Once again, I wondered, fleetingly, if doctors did that on purpose.

At the end of the examination, Dr. Wagner carefully explained that he could not make a judgment until he had a copy of the Mayo Clinic results and until he did some further testing himself. I explained the problem about getting the Mayo Clinic report locally, and that Dr. Madrid had sent to Rochester for it.

He told me he would approach Bill Collins for the report himself, and then assured me that he felt something was going on in my body. I had obvious muscle pain and the elevated sed rate and protein electrophoresis results suggested a collagen disease. He would know more after he had consulted with Dr. Collins and after he had done another battery of blood tests. He fussed over the fact that I was on Prednisone, telling me it was a dangerous drug for one thing, but more to the point, it could be masking important symptoms. We agreed for me to taper off it. Then, he told me to come back in two weeks to discuss the situation further.

It was difficult to read Dr. Wagner's reaction to me as he expressed so little emotion, but at least he had not dismissed me outright. I did not dare allow myself to hope that this man would finally come up with answers, so I firmly pushed him out of my mind. I had only gone to get Dr. Madrid off my back about the St. Louis business and to satisfy Dale. Dale simply would not let me quit. He was not pushing the St. Louis trip, but he did insist I see Dr. Wagner.

Two weeks later, I dutifully presented myself back in Dr. Wagner's office, and he gave me the results of his findings. My sed rate was still elevated, other blood tests were inconclusive, my physical symptoms were real but undefinitive, and yes, there was something wrong with me, but no diagnosis was possible at that time. He gave me a great deal of clinical information that went right over my head, assuming my limited medical knowledge was more extensive. I was almost flattered.

"It could be lupus," he said, "because the disease can smolder with discernible physical symptoms such as you are experiencing, for months, before any lab tests come back positive." He concluded by saying there was simply not enough evidence to make a diagnosis at that point in time. We would just have to wait and watch.

There it was. Lupus again.

He suggested I keep in close touch with Dr. Madrid, report to either one of them any further symptoms, and that he would contact Dr. Madrid regarding his findings.

I went back to my office at the university and called Dale to report in. It was a gloomy, rainy, fall day, unusual for the Southwest, but perfectly suited for the mood of the moment. Dale took the news in relative silence, and I could tell that even he was at a loss. We arranged for another session together later that week, and I hung up. I was, of course, discouraged, except for one small detail. Dr. Wagner was a most business-like person, reserved, even distant, yet he did ask me to promise him that I would call him the moment anything new or unusual developed. Beneath the professional veneer, I sensed a person who knew what he was doing, who was maybe interested and who, above all, believed me and possibly even cared.

CHAPTER NINE

OCTOBER, 1985

The period from late September after I had seen Dr. Wagner until the end of October when the final crisis began was a strange time for me. I had pretty much exhausted what the medical profession could do for me at the moment and even though Dale and Dr. Madrid and perhaps even Dr. Wagner were still interested, there was little they could do. Dr. Madrid went out of town for the month of September, so I lost his support, and even Dale's patience waned one day as he suggested to me that I had nothing more than an annoying but passing virus and that it was time to get on with it. He even told me he did not want to hear the word pain anymore, that we were going to have to find another term for it, like "discomfort."

"A rose my any other name...," I remarked cryptically, and added a scatological epithet for good measure.

He grinned, shrugged his shoulders, and said, "It was worth a try."

During this time, the disintegration nightmares returned, and I would wake up exhausted. I would spend the entire night searching for my Visa card which had been stolen, I dreamed regularly that my teeth were falling out, that my little toy poodle was constantly in serious danger and I could not help him, and I was again plagued by corpses that would not lie quietly in their graves. Increasingly I was driven to medical books and to the College of Nursing library at the university as I desperately tried to diagnose my own case. It was difficult, however, because I had so little information. I had been reduced to taking words off medical insurance forms, to reading my records upside down across doctors' desks, and then taking what I could and researching it on my own. From this dubious and imprecise method, I learned a great deal more about collagen diseases, the immune system, and autoimmune disorders. Along the way, I also learned a great deal about human anatomy, the myriad number of diseases that can plague us, and I was, as Dr. Wagner had pointed out, picking up a pretty good medical vocabulary.

One day when I was working with Dale, I mentioned to him that the left temporal pain got worse when I opened my jaw. He told me to open my mouth wide and when I did as I was told, a sharp pain, like a surge of electricity, shot up the side of my head. Dale got all excited, telling me he had picked up the spasm on his machinery. He insisted I see an oral surgeon about a possible mandibular joint (the large joint in your jaw) dysfunction. I refused. No way.

No more doctors. He turned his wheelchair around until he was facing me head on and said, "Pardon?" I never have been any good at staring down authority figures, so I went.

The surgeon was a nice young man and was impressed with my medical knowledge. He took x-rays of my jaws and teeth, which were normal. He told me that he was not writing me off as a neurotic, however. "Some people, that is the first thing you think about when they walk in. But not you," he said.

I was deeply appreciative. He said he had never met anybody with quite the same set of symptoms I had described, and that he was going to go home and get out his books. He was sorry that he could do nothing for me, however, and wished me luck. I could hardly wait to get home and call Dale to tell him there was nothing wrong with my jaw. I had not been interested in this doctor visit at all, knowing from the outset that he would find nothing. I had earned the right to gloat.

Physically, I did not feel any better, however. The symptoms still nagged at me and came and went with abandon. The headaches, general muscle pain and malaise continued, varying in intensity, and kept up a vicious cycle of illness and depression. The fatigue was the most draining, and I attempted to compensate for it by exercising again. I started going to the health club to push weights in an attempt to build up some muscle tone in my scrawny arms and legs. All I managed to do was to strain my neck and shoulder muscles and intensify the headaches. Dale was annoyed with me when I told him what I had been doing and put the health club off limits. Swimming was okay, but no weights. As had occurred that past spring, however, the exercise did no good, not even swimming. It took a tremendous effort to make myself go to the pool and I would leave feeling like a weakling. Whenever I went to the health club, in spite of Dale's interdict, I was shocked at what I looked like in leotards in all those mirrors--a female AIDS victim, scrawny and emaciated. Emotionally, I was at dead center, the *Ancient Mariner*'s sargasso sea. I felt lifeless, uncaring, dull, aimless, stupid, and often indulged in orgies of self-criticism and self-hatred. I was disgusted with myself and felt guilty for not being able to control my life, and for not doing my job. I was putting minimal energy into my teaching, and I had not written a word in over a year.

I did, however, develop a new symptom during this dead time towards the beginning of October. I looked at myself in the bathroom mirror one morning after I got out of the shower, and my face was lit up like a clown's; I had a vivid red rash that spread over my nose and across both my cheeks like a bad sunburn. LUPUS. In my wanderings through medical textbooks, I had discovered that a butterfly rash over the nose and face was a classic symptom of lupus. My stomach took another nosedive and then slowly knotted until I felt nauseated. I am, however, good at rationalization, so I dismissed the rash as a figment of my imagination when it disappeared an hour or so later. And each morning as it reappeared and then faded, it got easier to dismiss. I now began to reflect on the sun sensitivity problem Dr. Wagner had questioned me about. As far back as my late teens, I had noticed that whenever I sat out in the sun, I would break out in a terrible rash, like hives, on my arms, legs, and chest. It was ugly, but would disappear in a day or so, and the accompanying fatigue and nausea that I sometimes felt after a day in the sun I attributed to the excessive heat. I had never thought to mention this problem to my doctors until Dr. Wagner asked me about it. Then I remembered the bout I had had in Florida that past Christmas. From my reading, I now knew that sun sensitivity was another basic symptom of lupus, but I was still in the denial stage of what I sensed was to come, and dismissed the idea.

The watershed occurred on Friday, October 18. During the course of my second interview with Dr. Wagner, I saw that he had managed to get a copy of the report from the Mayo Clinic. He did not tell me about it, but I knew he had it in my file because I could see the letterhead upside down in the folder on his lap. By this time, I had become used to reading my own medical records, and I found myself being resentful that these records were not given to me as a matter of course. I walked out of his office determined to get my hands on that report. Why I did not just ask him for it, I will never know. Probably because I still believed I had no right to it, and did not really think he would give it to me. Anyway, I have lots of friends who call themselves Doctor (after all, Ph.D's carried the title of Doctor for centuries while physicians were little more than barbers and leeches), and after some plotting and with absolutely no sense of guilt, I wrote to the Mayo Clinic in early October and asked them to send my records to Dr.________, who was in reality an English professor and an accomplice.

I finally got my hands on the report that Friday, and it was not nice. I had already learned of their diagnosis in early August, quite by accident. They had sent me an itemized bill in late July, and had apparently also sent a copy to my insurance company. However, on the insurance copy, they had typed in the diagnosis. They had not included my social security number on the insurance copy of the bill, so the insurance company sent it to me to fill in. There, typed on the bottom, was "cervical tension myalgia and situational depression." Translated, that means the muscles in my neck hurt because of tension and I was depressed about it. I was furious on several counts. I was angry that they would send a diagnosis to my insurance company for every insurance clerk to see, but they would not send it to me. But I was even more angry at the trivialization of my illness. I do not know why I was so upset. I had expected something like this from the way Dr. Campbell had dismissed me. When I told a friend about it, he said, "I could have told you at least that. Why didn't you ask me? Then you could have paid me the awesome sum the Mayo Clinic charged!"

As I read through the report, I was amazed at the clinical disinterest with which Dr. Campbell reported on the various tests they had conducted. He summarized my medical history, reported on the physical examination and listed the laboratory data with no editorial comment. He concluded that I had no organic disease, that I probably would not accept that fact, that most of my symptoms were functional as opposed to organic, and that I needed pain management and psychiatric evaluation. The MMPI was even more devastating. It concluded that patients who displayed the profile I exhibited were prone to psychosomatic disorders, and that I was dependent, submissive, passive, self-centered and demanding, and lacking in insight.

"Dependent," I screamed! "On my two poodles?"

And how could I possibly be passive and submissive and still have a Ph.D., and have upheld a responsible administrative position in a State University?

And on whom did I make demands? I am not married and I have no children. And no insight? I teach literature, on the college level, for crying out loud. The profile was that of a stereotypical bored, middle-aged, suburban housewife in the midst of a mid-life crisis. The scenario was so far from the truth that I should have been amused. But I was not. I felt like someone had punched me in the stomach, and my legs became rubbery as I read and reread in utter amazement.

I must have gone over both reports twenty times. It was obvious to me that the MMPI results had sabotaged the Mayo Clinic doctors' assessment of my medical situation right from the very first day. It did not matter what I told them; thy simply were not listening. And they even ignored the evidence of their own lab results. I had known what was in the report; I had already figured it out from the way Dr. Campbell had acted that last day in Rochester and because Collins would not release it. I had also been tipped off by the elusive diagnosis on the insurance forms. But I was not prepared to see myself dismissed so clinically in print.

Sometimes as I read it, it made sense and sometimes not. I went to see Dale to get him to interpret the MMPI results for me, and he valiantly tried to soften the blow. He told me I had peaked above normal in categories one and three, which he had suspected. High readings in those categories were normal for a person in chronic pain, he explained. He told me the reliability factors on tests such as the MMPI were low, and in no case was it ever to be used as a diagnostic tool, as the Mayo Clinic doctors had obviously done, particularly without a psychological consultation with the patient. I sat in his office listening to about a quarter of what he was trying to tell me, not realizing that this final shock had pushed me over the edge of my ability to cope. I left in a daze, annoyed when he took off down the hall with one of the physical therapists without so much as a goodbye to me. At the time I felt he was being insensitive, but I now know the interview had been difficult for him, and he felt uncomfortable with what he had had to tell me.

After leaving Dale's office, I slowly and deliberately took the elevator to the main floor of the hospital, walked through the lobby to the front doors and left. Then, I walked out to the parking lot, got in my car, drove to the grocery store, shopped, and went home in a fog. After I got home, I began, mechanically, to clean my house in preparation for a party my teaching assistants had talked me into having that night at my house. At least I will have something else to think about, I kept telling myself, even if only for this one evening. And then about five p.m. the phone started ringing. This person could not come because she needed to stay home with her children and she knew I would understand, and that one was sick, and two others had found themselves dates which made for a more interesting evening; in other words, the party was off. That did it. The pain in my throat and chest which had been building all day came on in full force. I could not cry. I could get out an occasional dry, heaving, jerking sob, but that was it. When I am upset, I cry easily, and the release is usually healing. But not this time. I wandered around my house aimlessly, sat in the backyard for hours, went to bed for a time, woke up, wandered around some more, and on it went for two days. I was in some kind of a time warp where my surroundings did not make sense and time meant nothing. Usually I pick over my problems, analyze them, intellectualize them, ad nauseam, in an attempt to understand and come to terms with them. But this time I thought and felt nothing except the crushing pain in my throat and chest and gut.

I had some lucid moments. I remember making breakfast on Sunday morning, slowly and deliberately, but most of those two days is a total blank in my memory. I was in a state of almost complete self-hatred, utterly convinced that I was not a nice person, that I was a fake, self-centered and self-indulgent. Despite all the previous rationalizations over what the Mayo Clinic doctors had said about me, they had hit home, and at times I entertained the possibility that maybe their assessment of me was valid. Then I would switch sides and rage in self-pity at the medical profession in general and at the Mayo Clinic in particular. I got sick, I told myself, and went to them for help. They listened to me, took my money, subjected me to all kinds of cruel and painful treatment, lied to me, withheld information, mauled me, humiliated me, and then spit me out labeled "neurotic." In my imaginings, I even turned on Dale, railing at him and accusing him of being strident and flippant as he explained the MMPI results to me. These times of blame and name-calling and self-flagellation, as intense as they were, however, were nothing compared to the times when the dark whirlpools of pain and emptiness swirled around me. It was hard to breathe past the blockage in my chest, and when I took a deep breath to relieve the pressure, it came in jerks. And then there were moments when I started shaking and could not stop. And then the dead calm would come back and I would sit for hours doing nothing, thinking of nothing.

I tried to get out of bed on Monday morning to go to school, but every time I got up, I passed out. I made it as far as the bathroom on the third try and had to hold myself against the sink until the whirling dizziness passed. I managed to let my two dogs outside and then staggered back to bed. I called in sick, and I think I slept the entire day. David had heard from our departmental secretary that I kept fainting and called that evening to check on me. But whenever I tried to tell him what had happened, I was consumed with choking sobs. I was still not crying, only choking and dry sobbing. I could not talk to him and hung up the phone. He called back several times, but I did not answer. I could hear the phone off in the distance, ringing vaguely, not enough to demand my attention. I felt a strange calm, and wanted to try to tell him not to worry, that I was in control, but I couldn't talk. I went out into the backyard again, and as I wandered around among the trees, I felt a death wish gently flutter around my head and settle over my shoulders, softly, almost like a butterfly. Then, suddenly, my body became terribly heavy and I felt myself jerk into a new dimension where the only sound was a deadly, threatening, screaming ringing, like cicadas. I was, for a moment, terrified. I had never in my life been suicidal, preferring, like Hamlet, to bear those ills I had than to take on the unknown. This was an entirely new experience for me. Finally, I felt myself gibber and shudder as I was consumed by the uselessness of it all, even dying. I had given up, completely, but felt no relief as I gave up the struggle. I could almost physically feel myself fracturing into pieces, becoming disjointed, disoriented, yet possessed of a deadly calm, powerless to confront whatever it was that was possessing my body and soul.

It was my Catholic sense of responsibility and guilt, together with a mindless automatic and rote behavior, that got me out of bed the next morning. I had already missed one day of school and since I was not ill, I had better not miss another. I somehow managed to get myself dressed and to the university. I taught my Shakespeare class in a dream state, and I thoroughly impressed myself that I could walk into the room, take attendance, and conduct the class as if nothing had happened. I felt disembodied, the real me watching this puppet talk about *King Lear*, and doing it intelligently. I can also remember looking at the faces of my students and thinking they were not real. At one point, they blurred together, twenty moon-like shapes looking at me blankly, expectantly. I had never completely appreciated the surrealistic until this class.

When I got back to my office, my colleagues began to troop into my office, having heard from the departmental secretary that I had spent the previous day fainting, and from David that I had spent the evening in hysterics. Ruth had dropped by to talk to me about her Master's thesis and watched open-mouthed as person after person came in to express concern. In the middle of the parade, my father called from Florida. He informed me my mother had taken an early flight and that she would arrive that evening. Apparently, someone had called him, but I never discovered who. I assured Ruth I was not breaking down, although I knew I was, and got her out of my office. I called Dale, but he was out of town for the day. I was disappointed, but not inordinately so. There was nothing he could do. All the king's horses and all the king's men could not glue me back together again.

A friend drove me to the airport that evening, and as I greeted my mother, I was partly resentful, I felt silly, and I was enormously relieved at having her there. I did not trust myself, and I was afraid I would pass out again. After we got home, I told her about the Mayo Clinic report, the effect it had had on me, and that it had been the last straw. I described to her how I felt crushed, destroyed, annihilated as a person, angry, insulted, humiliated. I gave her both the letter Dr. Campbell had written and the MMPI results. She read them looking confused and shaking her head. I still did not know whether she was one hundred percent convinced that my problems were not emotional, and my current state of affairs certainly gave her reason to think that way.

During the three weeks she stayed with me, however, it became more and more obvious to both of us that there was something seriously wrong. I was utterly exhausted, all the time, and could barely drag myself to school to meet my classes. Her first order of business was to go out and shop for a couch for my office. "If you must work," she stated flatly, "at least this way you can lie down between classes." She was particularly distressed over my loss of weight, and was convinced that she had to stay to make sure I ate properly. She bought gallons of ice cream, made bran muffins full of nuts and raisins and dried fruits, poured butter into everything she cooked, and even filled my refrigerator with Metracal, insisting I drink it in addition to eating. She got that one from Larry. My weight problem was the least of my worries, trivial in comparison to the other symptoms I was suffering, but it gave her a focus for action, and she went after it with gusto. I tried hard to keep up a normal front as I visited with her, slept, went through the motions of my everyday routine, and just generally went on. Even when you are having a nervous breakdown and your health is slowly disintegrating, life does not stand still. One has to get up in the morning and do the mundane things of living. I often found myself curled up in my waterbed, my small poodle nestled against me, comforted by the domestic noises in the kitchen as my mother prepared meals or washed dishes. I suppose everyone is entitled to at least one trip back to the womb, and this was mine.

I finally tracked Dale down a day or so after my mother arrived, and when I told him over the phone that I had come unglued, he immediately cleared his schedule and made me come to see him that afternoon. I got to his office around three. He shut the door, wheeled around to face me, and gently asked what had happened. I blurted out in about three sentences that the TA party had collapsed the day we discussed the Mayo Clinic report and that I had spent the five days since we had last met having a nervous breakdown. He asked me a few pertinent questions, like whether I was crying uncontrollably and what happened when I took a deep breath. I told him I had not really been crying, only choking and sobbing, and when I took a deep breath, it came in jerks. Then he asked me if I would see a psychiatrist friend of his mainly because he thought I should be on medication to get through this crisis. I refused outright. I was not about to submit myself to yet another male doctor and to go through the authoritarian invasion of my person and my emotional privacy all over again. I may be many awful things but I am not stupid, I told myself.

Our conversation was jerky at first as Dale asked me simple questions and I blurted out answers. Gradually, however, I calmed down enough from the acute distress of having to admit to him that I was out of control, and started to talk more rationally. He asked me why I had reacted so violently to the Mayo Clinic's assessment of my character, and suggested maybe it was that the flaws they had pinned on me were the ones I most abhor. I readily admitted to that possibility, but actually it went far deeper, I told him. I have always had trouble admitting to my faults or accepting criticism. Indeed, in the ten months I had been seeing Dale I had skirted around any such discussions, believing they would diminish me in his estimation. I have always worked hard to present a controlled and together ethos to the world, and having to admit that I was less than the perfectly mature adult was humiliating to me. Consequently, I had hidden and repressed much from him, until now. The specific flaws the Mayo Clinic had flung at me stung, but I was far more devastated and outraged by the fact they had called me flawed at all. I had sought their help for my medical problems, not my emotional ones, I told myself. My personality was simply none of their business.

For the first time in our relationship, I began talking to Dale about feelings and fears, about the emotional effects my illness had had on me and about my suppressed and confused feelings over the way my doctors had treated me. Up until now, I had managed to hide behind my illness, to act as if the physical symptoms and a proper diagnosis were my only problem in life. Now that I had lost control of my natural reserve and the protective cover was gone, years of repressed anger and insecurity came gushing out, much to my surprise. I have always been a private person, finding it difficult to share my inner self with someone else, and even though I trusted Dale, I was still not at all comfortable talking to him so intimately.

I stayed with him until 4:25, slightly more in control than when I arrived, and once again surprised myself by the cool I managed to assemble as I taught my 4:30 graduate seminar. I kept going back to Dale every two or three days, and the intensity of the emotional upheaval gradually lessened, although I still could not cry. My outrage was intense, yet I could not legitimately indulge it because I did not know if the Mayo Clinic was really in the wrong. Once again they had taken away from me the right to be sick and to have any authentic feelings either about my illness or about the way they had treated me. I remember one day going in to see Dale at the hospital, and hesitating before entering the building. I felt guilty going in there taking up the staff's time, when the other patients around me in the hospital corridors and elevators were legitimately sick.

Ruth called one evening and told me Larry wanted to see me in his office. She had told him about the scene in my office and that I was badly upset over the Mayo Clinic report. I went to see him a day or so later. He motioned me to an examining room, sat me on a chair in the corner, pulled up another one facing me, and told me once again that I was not nuts. When I showed him my copy of the report, he read it and then flipped it back to me.

"You do not need psychiatric evaluation," he stated flatly. "You need to find out what is wrong with you."

He then asked me how I had managed to get my hands on that report, and I told him that was none of his business. "It was not hard to do," I informed him smugly. He was amused.

When we returned to the waiting room, my mother, who had accompanied me, also expressed her frustration and said she wanted to take me back to Florida to be with them.

"It won't help," Larry quickly replied. "She needs to work out her problems here." Then he gave me some anti-inflammatory samples, probably not knowing what else to do but feeling he had to do something, told me he suspected one of the autoimmune diseases, and invited me and my mother over to dinner the next evening. We went, and he watched my plate like a hawk. It was a delicious meal, Chinese food that Stephen (who at that time was an aspiring chef) and his mother had cooked. I made a valiant effort to eat, and as soon as I managed to get down what was on my plate, he ordered it to be filled again. I was deeply appreciative of Larry's concern, and I could sense his helpless frustration. He was reaching out to me the only way he could, and I was touched.

For the next three weeks, I struggled on at school, feeling weaker and more ill every day. I tried to put up a good front for my mother, but I was not very successful at it. At one point in time, she told me to cool it, that I was creating a bad impression at work, and that I should not tell anyone about my problems. I sure didn't need that piece of maternal advice, as well-intentioned as it probably was. I was feeling guilty enough on my own over my poor performance at school and the way my life was falling apart. Any anyway, it was far too late. Everyone already knew.

CHAPTER TEN

NOVEMBER, 1985

My mother left on Saturday, November 9. My father was alone in Florida and was not used to being on his own. My poor mother was torn between responding to his needs, and leaving me when she knew the crisis had not been resolved. She kept saying she would stay if I wanted her to, she could cancel her plane reservation, and my father would just have to cope. I did not want her to leave, but I knew my condition could carry on the way it was for months. I somehow had to learn to continue on my own. I was better emotionally, or at least I was sort of in control, and I did not feel my physical condition was bad enough to warrant her staying. The morning she left, I dragged myself out of bed to take her to the airport, overcome with yet another bout of fatigue. She cried when I dropped her off at "Departures," her motherly instincts telling her I was not yet well. And she was right.

I went home and slept all day, and by that evening I had a fever of 102 degrees. When I looked at myself in the mirror, I was shocked. I was pasty white, had deep, dark circles under my eyes, and I looked gaunt, almost skeletal. I canceled out on a dinner engagement for the evening, and went back to bed. I had become so conditioned to feeling terrible that it did not even occur to me to call the doctor. The fever persisted through Sunday, and on Monday morning I finally called Dr. Madrid. He told me to get myself over to his office at noon, which I did. Irene came with me as I was too ill to drive myself. My eyes felt like burning coals, every muscle in my body ached, and I felt terribly weak, on the edge of fainting. All I wanted to do was sleep. For once, Dr. Madrid saw me almost immediately, and when I walked in, he took one look at me, shook his head, and called Dr. Wagner to ask him what to do. They decided on blood tests, so I went over to the hospital and had them done.

In the blood lab, the technician told me they had to take blood every half hour for the next two hours. There were a couple of chairs in the hall where we could wait. The hall was dingy and the chairs were hard-backed kitchen chairs. This arrangement certainly would not do, as sick as I was. There was no way I could sit up for the next two hours in those chairs. I knew the hospital well, so I dragged Irene down the hall to the room where families wait while their relatives are undergoing surgery. I knew they had carpets and couches and soft music in there. I lay down on one of the couches and immediately went to sleep. I woke up with Larry standing over me. He had come in from surgery to talk to a family and had found me.

"What are you doing here?" he demanded.

Irene, who was sitting beside me reading, pointed out without lifting her head from her magazine, that I was sick again. Larry asked who was checking me out, and after I told him Dr. Madrid, he left, muttering to himself. I somehow managed to hang on for the two hours they needed for the blood tests, and then Irene took me home. I crawled back into bed without even undressing and went back to sleep.

Dr. Madrid called me that evening to tell me my white blood cell count was low, but that nothing else significant had shown up in the results that were in. He would call me when he knew more. As I hung up the phone, I noticed a new phenomenon. I felt as if army ants were crawling all over my body, and the itching and tingling were unbearable. Then Ruth called, Larry having told her he had run into me at the hospital, and suggested the tingling could be associated with the fever. The itching and the fever had somewhat abated by Tuesday morning, so I again went in to the university and taught my Shakespeare class. I am nothing else if not dedicated. As I was going down the hall to my class, one of my colleagues stopped me and told me I looked awful, that I needed to do something about it. I flew at him and shrieked, "What do you want me to do? Go to the doctor?!!" He backed off in a hurry. I went to bed Tuesday evening scratching at the "army ants" that had returned, feeling somewhat unreal, but glad the latest bout of illness seemed to be subsiding.

I woke up at two a.m. in agony. Waves of nauseating, sickening pain were driving through my chest, moving from the right side of the lower rib cage to the left. At first, I was terrified that I was having a heart attack, but I soon dismissed that idea because I could still breathe easily enough, when the pain let up between waves. I curled myself up in a ball and spent the remainder of the night alternately rocking on my elbows and knees and writhing around in the bed, whimpering, desperately trying to out-maneuver the pain. It was all-encompassing and took up my entire attention. I focused my total energies on outlasting the next crushing wave as it slammed through my chest, and when someone later asked me why I had not called for help, I replied I was too busy. That was not the real reason, however. Under any other circumstances, I would have recognized that I was in serious trouble and would have called for help. But I had been so brainwashed by the refusal of so many doctors to allow me to be ill that I did not behave as a sick person should and call for help, in spite of the acute distress I was suffering. The night was interminable. I slept fitfully, between attacks, and I found out that if I stacked four pillows behind me and sat upright in bed, the pain lessened somewhat. I could also control it by putting another pillow on my knees and doubling over it.

When morning finally came, the pain had abated somewhat and I could get to the kitchen to make some tea. As soon as the hour was decent, I put in a call for Dr. Wagner. Knowing Dr. Madrid's nocturnal habits, I decided there was no point in calling him that early. He was probably just getting home. I explained my problem to Dr. Wagner's nurse, and she told me to come to the office immediately. I slowly got dressed, and drove myself there. I even took my books with me prepared to go to the university after I had seen him. I still could not allow myself to be ill, as unbelievable as that might seem, and fully expected to be dismissed as undiagnosable once again. Dr. Wagner's nurse took me into one of the examining rooms, and I climbed up on the table, fully dressed, curled up in a corner, and dozed. When Dr. Wagner came in a few moments later he startled me awake. He heard my explanation, listened to my chest, sat down on one of those hard-backed chairs, and very quietly explained that I needed to go to the hospital immediately. I was not to go home to get my belongings, I was not to go to the university, I was to go directly to the hospital as soon as he had finished writing up some orders. Period.

The next few hours were a blur. I called Irene from a pay phone in the lobby of Dr. Wagner's building and asked her to come and bring me a housecoat and slippers. Then I walked to the hospital which was behind Dr. Wagner's office building and went to find Dale. He was dismissing a patient, and as soon as he had finished, he pulled me into his office, shut the door, turned his wheelchair around to face me, and told me I looked awful. I felt awful, and realized now that I was really sick. After I told him I was being admitted, I started to focus in on trivia and worried that I had nothing with me to wear. "We will give you something to wear," he promised me with a smile. "It opens in the back." Realizing that I was terribly frightened, he also assured me that they would not let me die and told me I had better go upstairs and check myself in. All I wanted to do was get into bed and go to sleep, so I left and dragged myself up to Admitting.

They were waiting for me with a wheelchair and even bypassed the usual admission routines. They took my insurance card and made a copy of it, placed a plastic identification bracelet around my wrist and ordered me into the wheelchair. When I protested that I could walk to the floor by myself, the admissions clerk firmly said, "Not to Telemetry you are not!" Telemetry is an intensive heart-care unit. As I was being wheeled into the elevator, a woman hospital worker standing in the rear remarked that it looked like trip to the hospital was interrupting a day at work. I was dressed in a gray woolen suit and had my briefcase in my lap. She touched my shoulder and told me she was sorry, without a trace of condescension. I was deeply impressed with her powers of observation and her true empathy for my situation. Not all medical people are bad guys, I said to myself. In less than ten minutes time I was flat in bed in the Telemetry Unit.

The first thing the nurses did, even before the usual history taking and urinalysis, was to hook me up to a portable heart monitor. They place electrodes on your chest, attached to a small receiving unit, about as large as a small cassette player. You carry it around with you wherever you go, and the nurses can constantly monitor your heartbeat from the nursing station. If anything goes wrong, an alarm goes off. Irene arrived with a housecoat and slippers and I arranged with her to deal with the practical affairs of this hospital stay, like getting my car out of the parking lot behind Dr. Wagner's building and taking it home, and packing me an overnight case with all the essential items one needs in a hospital. I also arranged for one of my teaching assistants to go and stay at my house and take care of my dogs. It is amazing how we focus in on the practical in a time of crisis. There must be some kind of innate human response that prevents us from panicking and killing ourselves. The nursing staff was exceptional. Everything they did to me they explained in detail, and nowhere was there ever conveyed to me a sense of urgency or impending trauma. They were quiet and cheerful, but firm, as they did things to me and gave directions.

Early that evening, after blood tests, an electrocardiogram, an echocardiogram, x-rays and other assorted hospital routines, Dr. Wagner appeared on the scene and told me they were uncovering all kinds of things. My white blood cell count was not just low, it was dangerously low, my sed rate had skyrocketed, and my liver enzyme readings were shockingly high. He was considering a liver scan and a bone marrow test but would wait overnight to see if the readings came down. I was to stay right where I was until he had some answers.

I was only too happy to stay where I was. The chest pains were starting to reappear, and I felt weak and nauseated again. When Dr. Wagner left, I got out of bed, and as I started to pace around the room to take my mind off the pain, I was beset with an entire range of conflicting and totally inappropriate feelings. I really was sick! There was indeed something wrong with me! And they were documenting it! I was intensely relieved, even exhilarated. But the sense of triumph and self-validation was immediately qualified by the burning sensation in my chest. My insides felt like they were on fire and the pain was shooting around the bottom of my rib cage, like exploding firecrackers. I felt terribly alone as the seriousness of what was happening to me gradually sunk in. I had been sick before, but I had never felt like this, never. I had wanted a label for my illness, something specific and tangible, and it looked like I would soon get what I wanted. As I stood at the window of my room, trailing the heart monitor and looking down at the lights from the city, I faced my own death, fully, for the first time in my life. It was a very real possibility now, maybe not tonight, but soon, just like it happened to other people. Overcome with a stinging loneliness, I got back into bed, curled up around my pain, and went to sleep.

I remained in the hospital until the following Sunday, November 17, a total of five days. The white blood cell count gradually came up and the liver reading came down. The chest pain slowly burned itself out and the "ants" went away as I began to feel better. One day Dr. Wagner informed me that my antinuclear antibody test had come back positive, with a high reading, that all these findings were pointing toward lupus, but he was not yet ready to accept that verdict until he had the results of more tests he had sent out of town. In the meantime, I was to rest and eat.

In addition to the regular meals, he ordered a snack to be sent to my room mid-morning, mid-afternoon, and each evening. It seemed that every time I turned around they were offering me something to eat, Jello in all colors of the rainbow, puddings, cookies, and anything with calories in it. I could not eat the regular meals, they were so terrible, so I called Ruth for help. She came by every day to visit, bringing hamburgers, delicatessen sandwiches, shortbread cookies, anything she could thing of to encourage me to eat.

Stephen came with her one day. He had found out the day I was admitted from a chance encounter on the street, that I was in the hospital with heart trouble. He charged over to the library to get his mother out of her study carrel, in an absolute panic Ruth reported to me, and then he called the hospital and had Larry paged. He made Larry find out what had happened and report back to him immediately. When Stephen came in my room, he demanded to know the diagnosis. I told him probably lupus. "Can they give you medicine to cure you?" he asked.

I told him, "No."

"Can they give you medicine to make you feel better?" he countered.

When I told him, "Yes," he threw back at me, "So what's your problem?" his obvious relief couched in the rigid and simplistic logic of a seventeen-year-old.

Larry also dropped by one day after surgery, concerned at my condition, but as smug as he could be when I told him Dr. Wagner was suspecting lupus. Dale came in the day after I was admitted and told me I looked much better than the day before. When I asked him if it was okay for me to be sick now, he smiled and said, "You're allowed." He was more relaxed than I had seen him in months, relieved that we were coming up with some answers, and that it was no longer just him and me against the rest of the world.

I went home that Sunday, in control of myself for the first time in a year and a half. Yes, there was something seriously wrong with me, as I had known all along, but now they were hearing me. I was not quite so alone with my anguish, and when my friends dropped by my house during the following week as I was convalescing, they no longer avoided looking at me directly. My mother and father arrived from Florida, having barrelled down the highway in two and a half days, thoroughly frightened for me, but this time there was a difference. We were finally getting answers, specific physical ones, which we could all deal with. The vague, drifting symptoms I had been experiencing all these months were finally coming together into something concrete that was acceptable to talk about, as bad as it was. I saw Dr. Wagner in his office on Friday, November 22, and he quietly and at length went over all my test results with me and told me I had systemic lupus erythematosus. He gave me the bottom line as he told me the disease was potentially life-theatening, but not necessarily so, and we discussed a program of therapy. I walked out of his office light-headed, relieved, dazed, and with a sense of unreality. When I saw Dale later that day and told him, he reacted quietly. He did not have all that much to say; he just took notes, and sighed a lot, and told me to do the things at work that I really liked.

CHAPTER ELEVEN

COPING

Only gradually, over the next several weeks, was I able to internalize and accept what was happening to me. The initial and overwhelming sense of relief I experienced, as absurd as it might appear, is a normal one for patients who go through a long history of frustration in obtaining a diagnosis. Such patients usually become much more quickly adjusted to their illness than do those who experience a sudden onset of disease, mainly because they have already lived with it, sometimes for years. Once my doctors legitimized my illness, I accepted, indeed embraced, the sick role with gratitude. I could now act as a sick person should, and when Dr. Wagner told me I was not to go back to work for another week, I did not object nor did I feel even a trace of guilt.

The glorious indulgence of languishing in the hospital, being pampered and catered to and feeling vindicated was short-lived, however. These feelings soon gave way to a series of reactions I have since come to understand are normal for a person given a prognosis such as mine.[1] As soon as I was out of the hospital and knew for certain I had lupus, I experienced a gut reaction that terrified me. I was sure I was going to die, despite Dr. Wagner's reassurances. I became obsessed with the ghoulish aspects of death. I read obituaries in the paper, and whenever I drove past a cemetery I felt a sense of inevitability and resignation. I gave up planning for my future as a professor, as a person, and for a time lived completely inside the present. Then I began to think my life had been wasted, that I had not yet had time to accomplish anything important, and now never would. I also experienced a touch of the absurd. Although life and death are of tremendous significance as a general concept in our society, any one person's life can end with barely a stir. I realized my passage would not be all that earth-shattering, apart from affecting those few people immediately close to me. The university would go on doing its business without giving me a second thought, and I would go on record merely as another lupus statistic. Surely there was more to life than this. I was obsessed with such morbid thoughts, and I could not bring myself to discuss these fears with anyone, not even Dale.

Even now, years later, I still think a great deal about dying. That first night in the hospital when I suspected I had lupus, I reached an irreversible

[1]See Robert H. Phillips, *Coping With Lupus* (New Jersey: Avery Publishing Group, 1984), Part II.

awareness of my own mortality that has never left me, an awareness that now colors everything I do. Death touches our lives at every turn, so I have discovered, if we choose to see it. Most of us, however, particularly when we are young, avert our gaze from death, and perhaps rightly so. Ibsen was quite right when he observed that human kind can bear only so much reality.[2] To live in the constant shadow of death is paralyzing and inimicable to progress. But we all must, at some time, face it. As Norman Cousins put it, "The ultimate truth about life is that it is transient," and serious illness brings this truth home as nothing else can.[3] I have not yet come to Cousins' peaceful acceptance of the inevitable, however. In the years since I have been diagnosed, I have become used to the idea of my own death, but I am not yet resigned to it.

Apart from the fear of dying, a sentence of chronic illness makes one face the possibility of a loss of independence and all the humiliations that accompany that terrible state. I felt this loss acutely. My independence is something I take great pride in and treasure. I have always done things for myself, earned my own living, taken care of my own house and garden, made my own life-decisions, and I was desperately afraid that I would soon become dependent on other people and that I could not live by myself anymore. I often take my dogs to nursing homes with the Pet-a-Pet program and feel keenly the loneliness and humiliation and loss of self-hood the inmates live with daily. My mother and father stayed with me for a couple of months after I knew I had lupus and took complete control of my house and my life. They did the shopping, drove my car, cooked meals, and even told me when to go to bed. Although they meant well and I needed their help, they inadvertently contributed to my fears.

I have had many ups and downs since that first serious attack, but so far have managed to remain self-sufficient. I still experience chronic fatigue and weakness, nausea, rashes and severe headaches, and, in addition, I have developed arthritic pain in my hands and hips. I also suffer from repeated abdominal distress caused by an immunosuppressant drug, Imuran that I now take. Finally, as a result of the long-term use of Prednisone, I have recently had two cataract operations, and I have trouble controlling my weight. While none of these conditions has seriously threatened my freedom, they have certainly qualified my life style and serve as a constant reminder of what is possible. I continue to be hospitalized with recurrent flares once a year or so, and each one is a stunning reminder to me of the fragility of good health and the potential for losing control over one's life. At a recent gathering of friends where one had rheumatoid arthritis and another multiple sclerosis, both women admitted that their greatest fear is not dying, but becoming so incapacitated that they will have to depend on others for their well-being. Indeed, nothing circumscribes one's life so severely as chronic illness.

Even though I am not immediately threatened by a serious loss of my independence, I still suffer from another bane of chronic immune system disorders, overwhelming fatigue and weakness. Such weakness is soul-draining and utterly destructive of one's normal life. Flannery O'Conner referred to her lupus as the "energy draining disease," and I know what she meant.[4] I have

[2]*The Wild Duck*

[3]Norman Cousins, *The Healing Heart*, 230.

[4]Flannery O'Connor, *A Habit of Being: Letters of Flannery O'Connor*, ed. Sally Fitzgerald (New York: Farrar, Straus, and Giroux, 1978).

told my friends that I tire easily and that I will often have to leave an evening's gathering early, or not come, but they still become impatient with me. Some of my friends with chronic illnesses tell me they have great difficulty with their husbands who simply cannot understand why they are completely debilitated one day, and fine the next. One woman I know with multiple sclerosis attempted to suppress her physical exhaustion and to keep up an even pace with her husband. She only succeeded in destroying her health and, ultimately, her marriage. In my own case, I can feel the resentment when I back off from a committee assignment or do not attend meetings at work. It is difficult for any ill person to decide when to keep one's ills to oneself and when to communicate them as an appropriate explanation for not doing something. The months I was dismissed as neurotic have had a permanent effect on me, and I am now supersensitive to my weakness and debilitation being interpreted as whining or goldbricking. Consequently, I often find myself going places or doing things I should not. I also find it difficult to tell others when I need support, particularly in the times of fatigue and the inevitable depression that accompanies it.

One of the most common results of the above conflicting pressures is anger, and I have certainly experienced my share. Many people simply cannot understand why they have been singled out with the burden of long-term illness and rage at those close to them, at themselves, at their doctors, at the gods. Indeed, it has often been observed that it is not just the patient who is stricken with cancer, or rheumatoid arthritis, or whatever disease, but the entire family. I am not angry that I have lupus, because it is no one's fault, nor do I feel this illness has been visited upon me by an avenging God for my past sins. A curious combination of genetic factors and environmental stress probably caused the lupus to emerge, but I now suspect I have had it all my life. I have always been tired, I had suspected rheumatic fever as a child which was probably lupus, and I have had repeated bouts of pneumonia and respiratory infections throughout my adulthood, all probably lupus-related. The diagnosis of lupus was not a new experience for me, but merely a discovery of what had been going on for a very long time. My personal burden of anger, then, is not disease-related, but is directed at those members of the medical profession who refused to accept me as a credible witness to my own illness.

Nor am I alone in this anger. Until the advent of blood testing into DNA which has just come about in the last couple of years, most patients with lupus suffered the same distress in their search for a diagnosis as I did, some much, much worse. When I first started attending lupus support group meetings, I was humbled by some of the shocking horror stories I heard of others who had likewise been mauled by the medical profession. One woman admitted it took her ten years to finally find out she had lupus. And I constantly read in newspapers and magazines of cases where an individual was dismissed by doctor after doctor as neurotic, only to finally discover she had some long-term chronic illness. It is difficult to deal with the resulting anger that comes from this kind of rejection.

Another ramification of chronic illness is isolation and depression. Serious illness sets the patient apart from other people, and as much as one's family and friends care, there is nothing much they can do. In the end, it is the individual's asthma, or lupus, or multiple sclerosis, or scleroderma, or whatever, and it is the individual who must accept it and learn to live with it.

But it is difficult, especially with some of the chronic immune disorders. For the most part, the ravages of these diseases go on inside the body, with little external evidence. People find it difficult to be sympathetic to a person who is ill but who looks healthy. Those who have heard of lupus, for example, think it is terminal and usually blurt out their misgivings. "That's fatal!" gasped the boyfriend of Irene's granddaughter upon hearing of my affliction. And of course my literary friends are fond of pointing out that Flannery O'Connor died of lupus. Phillips calls this the big mouth syndrome.

Perhaps the most difficult ramification of serious illness, however, is depression. Most of the literature on illness-related depression explains it as reactive, a natural anger and sense of betrayal that really has no object. Most people go through a grieving process at the profound sense of loss, particularly at the lack of being able to do things formerly done with ease. For example, for younger lupus patients (ninety-five cent are young women), not being able to go to the beach and tan represents a serious loss. For me, my lack of energy and constant need for sleep is a source of frustration. Marriages and long-standing relationships suffer from the ravages of the withdrawal and depression that almost always accompanies chronic illness, and the usual dynamics of family life often have to change dramatically.

Any of the above events can cause acute depression, but I also think it can be explained in terms other than situational or merely reactive. Malcolm Rogers calls the kind of depression that is common to chronically ill patients "endogenous depression," a complex internal state spontaneously occurring, marked by feelings of hopelessness, helplessness, worthlessness, and global loss of pleasure.[5] Many chronically ill patients I have talked to describe this depression as their most wearisome burden, probably because it is so hard to control and comes without warning. Usually, there is no single adverse circumstance as a precipitating factor to explain another bout of the "blues"; it just happens, and is thoroughly debilitating. Many are now beginning to speculate that the chemical changes that are occurring in the body with the ravages of disease alter the delicate balance in the brain and so cause this kind of depression. This possibility is even more pertinent in the case of immune-related disorders as the immune system is so complex and all-encompassing in body processes. It is important that the patient understand all these factors and not blame herself, nor be scolded and blamed by others.

The behavioral science profession is now beginning to understand the psychological ramifications of long-term illness and is beginning to address the needs of such patients. Pain clinics have sprouted up all over the country, and, more and more, psychotherapists are specializing in the treatment of the chronically ill. Further, support groups along the lines of Alcoholics Anonymous are being formed nation-wide to meet the specific needs of people with such diseases as lupus, arthritis, AIDS, and cancer, and many religious groups are sponsoring retreats focusing on wellness therapy.

Most of these movements were in their infancy, however, when I was first diagnosed in 1985. After the initial euphoria of being vindicated wore off, I

[5]Malcolm P. Rogers, "Phychiatric Aspects," in *The Clinical Management of Systemic Lupus Erythematosus*, ed. Peter H. Schur, M.D. (Orlando, Florida: Grune & Stratton, Inc., 1983), 195.

was still left with my disease, and I still did not feel well. My depression returned with a vengeance, and at first I thought much of it was in response to the reactions of my family and friends. Although still supportive, they gradually returned to their own lives, relieved that the "problem" had been solved. For me, however, the problem had not been solved. I still had lupus, and I still did not feel well. At first I was angry at what I considered a betrayal, but then I came to understand that the lupus was, after all, my problem, and that I was the one who had to come to terms with it. Also, I misjudged some of my friends. I complained to a female colleague one day that I felt deserted, that no one would talk to me any more about my illness, and that I felt alone and isolated with my misery. Her answer took me completely by surprise and taught me a well-needed lesson in humility. "It is hard for us, too, you know," she said quietly.

At that point I realized I needed to develop my own coping strategies, so I began with the traditional sources of help, religion and therapy. Although I come from a devout Roman Catholic background, I had long ago given up on organized religion as having anything to offer me, mainly because of its teachings on human sexuality and its attitude toward women. Now, however, the potentially life-threatening nature of my illness forced me to contemplate the ultimate issues of the meaning of life and death, issues traditionally addressed in a religious context. At first, I experienced a sense of comfort and renewal when I re-embraced the formal religion of the Catholic Church, but I soon realized not much had changed. I had thought I could overlook those things that repelled me about the human side of the visible church, and to take solace in its ritual. But it wasn't enough. I simply could not get by its doctrinal arrogance and institutionalized sexism. I was in agonies of guilt and frustration when I had a dream that explained the solution for me:

> Someone brought in a fishbowl full of exotic fish. The bowl shattered with a bang in my hands. Tiny fish were flopping everywhere and I tried to rescue them. Then, someone brought in another bowl with two ordinary goldfish in it but I was not all interested. I returned to the task of trying to rescue the exotic fish; but they had escaped into a clear stream and were running free. I tried with a paper cup to scoop them up, but to no avail. Then, the idea of a fish net struck me, but I gave it up.

The fish is an ancient symbol of spirituality, one widely used by the early Christians. The bowl is, of course, the structure of the Church from which the exotic fish escaped. It is a suitable container for the ordinary goldfish (most people??) and they are happy in it, but apparently I identified with the exotic fish who longed to swim free. This dream taught me that I needed to forge my own personal spirituality, to be responsible for the salvation of my own soul with all the fears and confusions that would bring. But the reward is freedom to express my own spiritual needs in ways that are meaningful only to me.

Although I gradually accepted this spiritual insight, I still felt lonely and in need of human comfort and guidance. So I turned to the second standard answer, therapy. The psychological effects of having a serious illness--depression, anxiety, fear, anger, frustration, uncertainly--were too much for me to handle on my own, and the genuine, if unspoken, support from my friends was simply not enough. Dale was involved in biofeedback and a new pain clinic he was organizing, so I began seeing another therapist, mainly to talk through my fears and anxieties at being chronically ill, but more so to explore what I could legitimately expect of myself and of those around me in terms of support. With help, I learned to listen to my body, and now, when it signals "fatigue," I let it rest. Gradually, I learned to cope with the guilt and frustration at spending so much time in bed, and the "I should be's" have slowly dropped out of my vocabulary. I have discovered that if I fight the weakness and fatigue, that if I go on about my life in spite of the chronic debilitation, I only make things worse, get frustrated and uptight, and spend a great deal of time spinning my wheels. Now, if I have to rest three days of the week, I do it without feeling guilty and buy myself productivity the other four. Through the combined program of drug treatment and the conscious acknowledgement of and respect for my limitations, the payoff has been long periods of remission and a renewed sense of well-being.

Therapy, then, helped me to listen to my body and to obey its needs without guilt. But I also learned something far, far more valuable. My therapist was interested in dreams and encouraged me to keep a dream journal as a way of getting in touch with my inner self. I had always been skeptical of dream interpretations and resisted at first, but as I paid more attention, I was amazed at the workings of my unconscious. One dream in particular made me realize there really was something to this business. I can remember I was in one of my "well" periods, probably the result of a steroid rush. I had energy, appetite, and even felt like working. Life was suddenly good again. Then, one night I dreamed I was walking in a wooded area, the sun gently filtering through the trees. Behind many of the trees were wolves, not threatening, but sitting up and dozing in the sun, like dogs do when they are alert but feeling comfortable and secure. I took the dream to my therapist and we played with it for some time, but could make no sense of the message. Then, as I was driving home, it suddenly dawned on me. Lupus is the Latin word for wolf. An imaginative nineteenth-century scientist had first named the disease "lupus erythematosus," seeing the characteristically red (*erytheme* is Greek for "to be red") and ugly rash on the face of its victims as similar to the bite of the wolf. The other metaphoric connotations that surround the wolf--destructive, wily, predatory, rapacious--are also apt descriptions of the disease as it attacks its victim. The dream was clearly conveying to me that while dozing, the wolves were still lurking behind the trees, and I needed to respect that.

Fascinated, I began to pay more attention to my dreams and to my inner voice. I began to realize that my unconscious always signalled to me when a flare was approaching, usually through such dream images as my house developing huge cracks, or actually disintegrating and falling in thousands of tiny pieces on my head. One time I was in a room with the floor covered with broken glass that I was desperately trying to clean up, and in another I opened the front door and three large German shepherds (wolf-like in appearance) came charging into my house. The most impressive dream, however, occurred one night during a particularly bad flare and a series of excruciating headaches. I had raged and cried at the pain all evening and had finally drifted into an exhausted sleep when the dream came:

> I was sitting on the floor in my kitchen killing moths under the sink with my shoe. I had quite a pile going when suddenly a huge butterfly landed on my head. I could feel its claws on my scalp, like an eagle's. I didn't want to kill it; it was too beautiful. So I lifted up the window and gently tilted my head to let it fly free. Then, just as it was leaving, I lost my grasp on the window, and it slammed shut, crushing the butterfly in one corner.

I have a vivid picture, even now, of the window that had slammed shut and the upended and mangled body of the insect.

Again, I took my dream to my therapist and again we could make no real sense of it. Then, as had happened with the wolf dream, the meaning hit me with a lightening flash of insight. The Lupus Foundation uses the butterfly for its logo, partly because its transforming properties as it changes from the worm-like caterpillar into the beautiful adult butterfly signify hope, but more practically because the butterfly rash on the face and nose of the victim is so common a trademark of the disease. It was the lupus that was crushing my head, and yet I had a perverse attachment to my pain. I wanted to let the butterfly go free, but inadvertently destroyed it, as I let the window slip. I called my doctor the next morning, and he decided it was time to get aggressive with the drug therapy in order to crush this particular flare.

My struggles with chronic illness and all its attendant miseries, then, have not been an entirely negative experience. Both the search for a diagnosis and the years of coping since have been a psychological and even spiritual journey as well as a medical one. I have learned a great deal about medical matters, about other people and about inner resources for coping that I had no idea I possessed. In particular, I have noticed a phenomenon that is apparently not at all unusual for someone who has been through a serious illness. I have discovered that I have a heightened awareness of life, of its sorrows as well as its pleasures. The painful things I feel more keenly that I used to. I discovered this at a friend and colleague's funeral several months after I knew I had lupus. I felt her loss more acutely than I had ever imagined I would. It still hurts to think of her sudden death. On the other hand, I enjoy the simpler pleasures such as sunsets, and my rose garden, and dinner with a good friend, much more intensely. It is like living life in vivid color, rather than black and white.

All of the above is not to say I am glad for my lupus. I would get rid of it tomorrow, if I could, with no regrets. I suppose we all have to cope with what life deals us, each in our own way. I have learned that such coping is an essentially alone endeavor, which is the down side; but the up side is learning to cherish life because it is so precious and fleeting, indeed, to truly "seize the day."

CHAPTER TWELVE

BEING ILL IN AMERICA

The foregoing account of my sixteen-month search for a diagnosis of lupus and the gradual evolution of coping strategies I have developed since represent an attempt to contextualize my personal experience in the universal crucible of serious illness. Many writers have attempted to research the various psychological, economic, and social components of serious illness, but such studies inevitably do violence to what is essentially an organic, interdependent experience. Sociological studies of patient attitudes in the hospital, for example, come nowhere near capturing the fear, and loneliness, and physical pain, and humiliations, and anxiety and anger over what all this is costing. Only living through the agonies of prolonged illness can give one a taste of what it is to be immersed in a sea of conflicting feelings and social pressures, which is why I have chosen the first person narrative in tackling this difficult subject. I know I was often lost and angry as I attempted to piece together my fragmented life, but I emerged out of the chaos, maybe not a better person, but certainly a more knowledgeable one. To that extent, my experience represents a *felix culpa*. By way of conclusion, then, I would like to offer some final insights I have come to on this business of being ill.

i

To begin with, let us consider the health-care system and its role in the ill person's life. Ostensibly, it is there to ease pain, and to prolong life. But as my story vividly illlustrates, the system can also do much damage. Some of the reasons, in my particular case, can be attributed to the elusive nature of my disease; but not all of it. Nor do I think that my experience was an isolated aberration of medicine, or mere bad luck. Many people have approached me informally at parties, and even formally in my office, having heard of my nightmare and wanting to share their own unhappy medical encounters. They talk of their doctors not knowing what they were doing, of not having time to talk to them, of charging outrageous prices, of missing diagnoses, and, above all, of not believing them. Most self-help groups such as the American Lupus Foundation often arrange informal discussions at their meetings so participants can vent and hopefully purge their anger at the many doctors they claim have mismanaged them. This benign anger often turns ugly and more overtly hostile when there have been serious bunglings on the part of some doctors, especially surgeons. Witness the tremendous surge in lawsuits and the escalating malpractice insurance premiums that are now part of everyday American life.

Some of this suing can indeed be frivolous, motivated by simple greed as doctors are quick to point out, but much of it is not. Doctors are being sued, called to account some would say, by a more educated and informed clientele, people who are no longer content to do as the doctor says in ignorant trust and to accept complications as simply unfortunate. Part of the reason for this new assertiveness can be accounted for by the generally higher level of education on the part of the American public than what existed in the 1940's, but perhaps an even more important reason is the new consumerism that has finally reached medicine. For Cousins, the most important thing that has been happening in health care today is the fact that people no longer take products and services for granted.[1] Nor should the physician be threatened by this legitimate demand for accountability, he concludes. The new consumerism "can be an important source of the physician's support and growth, for what it is actually doing is seeking the best in the physician, even as the physician seeks to bring out the best in the patient."[2]

Many doctors, unfortunately, have reacted to this new demand for accountability with anger and hostility, sometimes refusing to treat a patient whom they suspect will be litigious, sometimes refusing to work in a particular specialty at all. Their common complaint is that we, as patients, expect too much of them and that we do not have a realistic appreciation of the limitations of modern medicine. They certainly have a point. I have often been amazed at the ignorance of some of my friends about the most basic facts concerning their own bodies and about common diseases. I have also been amazed at their blind trust in doctors on the one hand, and their intolerance of even the slightest uncertainty or mistake on the other. In their defense, medicine as a discipline fosters this kind of dependency with its rigid control of information, its mysterious language and its intimidating machines. But we as patients must learn to confront and challenge this barrier, to be responsible and informed patients, and to become more in charge of our own medical care.

And there are many ways we can do just this. To begin with, it is absolutely imperative that we, as patients, learn more about the workings of our bodies, about disease, and about medications. Many have told me that I am not the usual patient, that I have a Ph.D, that I have learned to read in many disciplines and to find my way easily around a library. I cannot accept this line of reasoning. Most people out there learn to do their own taxes, learn to do basic car repairs, and figure out how to operate their home computers. Surely they can learn the basics of medicine they way they have learned about economics, mechanics, and word processing. Many good books are available for the lay reader, and every Sunday I read in the morning paper about local hospitals offering courses and workshops in diabetes, rheumatism, alcoholism, kidney diseases, stress management. In addition, many communities now have a community college and it would behoove all of us to take a course in cardiopulmonary resuscitation, in general first aid, or in basic anatomy. I simply cannot

[1]*The Healing Heart*, 159.
[2]P. 166

buy the argument that all medical knowledge is beyond the reach of the average citizen. The medieval clergy fostered the same myth about theology, that it was too refined and esoteric for vulgar minds, and in order to maintain control, to keep themselves as the sole interpreters of truth, they kept the language of theology in Latin. William Tyndall, the first man to translate the Bible into English, was burned at the stake as a heretic, when all he was attempting to do was to demystify theology and to make the mysteries of faith accessible to all.

In addition to knowledge, we patients also have an obligation to keep our bodies healthy and disease-free by such practices as exercise, good nutrition, by not smoking, and by drinking moderately. Further, we need to learn to participate in medical encounters as adults, to ask questions about the side effects of drugs, about the necessity of tests and treatments, and if necessary, to insist on seeing the results of laboratory tests and reports. Szasz and others divide the physician-patient encounter into three distinct categories: (1) active/passive, or the parent/infant model appropriate to the critically-ill emergency case; (2) guidance/cooperation, or the parent/child relationship where the patient is trustful and the physician has most of the say; and (3) mutual participation or the adult/adult relationship.[3] We would all like to think we operate in the last category, but few of us do. We need to be careful not to allow the doctor to put us in the parent/child relationship, and if he does, we need to drop him. Many of us fall into the trap of not wanting to bother the doctor because he is too "busy" with more seriously ill patients, or that he has many more demands on his time than we do. Doctors are only as busy as they allow themselves to be, and they are well-compensated for their time. We need to remember that we are paying for his or her services, and we have a right to careful attention. We are the consumer, and we need to hire our doctors the way we would hire a lawyer or a garage mechanic, as fee for services. One of the worst traps patients fall into is to let the doctor intimidate them and to let their personal concern for his feelings get in the way of a second opinion or a direct question.

Finally, patients need to keep a file of their own medical records, to take notes after they have visited the doctor, to record dates of immunizations and illness episodes, to made records of drugs taken and their efficacy, and to record dates of all surgeries, no matter how minor. The greatest misconception that most patients harbor is that their doctor "knows their bodies" and has complete and accurate records of their medical history. What I am saying, once again, is that we as patients must learn to take charge of out own health care by being knowledgeable and responsible consumers.

Doctors, on their part, must also learn to change certain attitudes and behaviors. They could begin by arranging physical space in their offices, in hospitals, in clinics, so it is more patient-centered. Such simple matters as waiting rooms that are large enough to handle the number of patients, comfortable chairs arranged appropriately, and sensible scheduling to minimize waiting time would be a good place to start. I just came from a recent doctor's appointment where I had to wait for an hour and a half to see the doctor. It was not an emergency that called him away, nor was it even a full waiting room that had caused him to be behind schedule. Just before he got to me, he decided to take

[3]See Anderson and Helm, "The Physician-Patient Encounter" in Jaco, *Patients, Physicians and Illness*, 260.

a break, and went upstairs to a lounge area to rest. I heard the nurses discussing the matter in the room next to me while I cooled my heels in the examining room. That kind of behavior is the height of arrogance.

Nor would it be inconceivable for hospitals to modify their behavior to put the patient first, not the staff. Simple courtesies such as knocking before entering the patient's room, and not barging into the room and asking about bowel functions in front of the patient's visitors would do wonders for the patient's sense of self-respect. And surely, schedules could be arranged so that patients are weighed in the middle of the day, when they are normally awake, not in the middle of the night. And I see no reason why hospitals could not set aside an area on each floor, for patients who are well enough, to congregate and to socialize. Illness is a frightening experience, and patients could gain much support from each other if they were allowed to communicate.

Medical workers also need to train themselves and their employees to recognize and to eliminate the language of condescension and subjugation that is so ubiquitous in health-care settings. I was indulging in a parody of such language one day for the benefit of my family, pulling out such phrases as "Step up here for me, dear," or, "Now if you can just swallow this for me," or, "This won't hurt a bit; there, see now. It's all over." My father was incredulous. He admitted he had never been treated that way, but then, being a white, male, executive type, he is high on the scale of those who get respectful and humanized care. Another major way health-care workers employ language to control is to shut the patient out from the talk. Doctors generally are much more open to the patient's family than to the actual patient, and they often congregate in the hallway outside a patient's hospital room to confer with family members, not in the room in front of, and including, the patient. And doctors consult with one another about a particular course of treatment for a patient and then merely inform the patient what they have decided.

Perhaps the most infuriating and controlling practice in American medicine is to deny patients access to their medical records. Just about anyone in the hospital, from the medical director to the lowliest lab technician can see these records, but not the patient. Upon being discharged from the hospital one time, I upset the entire floor by asking for a copy of my records before I left. The shock and concern on everyone's face was so remarkable, I left without them, vowing to return when I felt better. I presented myself to the records department about two weeks later and filled out a form requesting my records. In the space asking for the reason for the request, I wrote in "personal." You would have thought I was trying to infiltrate the Pentagon. All kinds of people came out and asked why I wanted them. After many hushed consultations behind various partitions, the supervisor finally came out and told me there would be a fifty-dollar fee and then a one-dollar-a-page charge to photocopy my records. When I sputtered that I had already paid handsomely for these records in the ten-thousand-dollar bill they had sent me for my hospital stay, she responded that the charge was to discourage people from making such a request. So I lied and said I wanted to consult with an out-of-town physician and needed to take the records with me. She capitulated, and gave them to me, but only the lab results, not the doctor's reports. When I asked a doctor friend about the paranoia in making doctor's reports available, he responded they did not want to be held accountable for all their written notes. When I pointed out that these "written notes" became a permanent part of a patient's records, and maybe if they were readily available, doctors would be more responsible in what they wrote down, he just shrugged.

The mindset that would make such information privileged is something I simply cannot understand. Yes, patients are much more docile if the doctor controls the information, but they certainly cannot participate in their own care if they do not understand what is going on. It doesn't take long to explain to a patient what lab results mean. It should be standard practice for all labs in the country to send a copy of any tests directly to the patient, as well as to the doctor. After all, it is the patient who pays for them. When we hire a lawyer and pay him or her handsomely to find out information for us, would we tolerate it if he or she decided to hold back in case the information would upset us, or maybe we would not understand it?

Another serious problem ubiquitous in the medical profession is the instinct to stereotype. Once again, the sociological literature on doctor-patient dynamics suggests doctors are much influenced by a patient's age, race, sex, physical appearance, occupation, far more than they realize.[4] For example, two studies that were recently published in the *The New England Journal of Medicine* suggest there is some pernicious sexism endemic to medical care. According to the studies, women who are hospitalized for coronary heart disease undergo fewer major diagnostic and therapeutic procedures than do men. The researchers conclude such findings "may represent a sex bias in the delivery of medical care."[5] The ramifications of such biases are shocking and far-reaching, for at the very least they suggest the bias against women may have been institutionalized into every corner of medical treatment. And it has been well-documented in the literature that male patients are taken more seriously and are more readily believed than are female patients.

Finally, and perhaps most important, is the problem of communication. I often fuss at my freshman composition students for writing with what I call the "egocentricity of the writer"; that is, they write with no concern for the needs of their reader. They know the subject, and they know what they are trying to say, but they often do not understand, much less consider, that their discourse has to be adapted to the needs of the particular audience they are addressing. My greatest challenge as a teacher of writing is to make my novice writers produce "reader-centered" prose. The same principles hold true for doctor-patient communications. Patients often give a garbled, incoherent, and incomplete history to their doctors and then expect their physicians to make sense of their account, of their symptoms, and to make a one hundred percent accurate diagnosis one hundred percent of the time. Doctors, on their part, often assume an

[4]See Anderson and Helm, "The Physician-Patient Encounter," and S.W. Bloom, *The Doctor and His Patient: A Sociological Interpretation* (New York: Russsell Sage Foundation, 1963).

[5]John Z. Ayanian, M.D. and Arnold M. Epstein, M.D., "Differences in the Use of Procedures Between Women and Men Hospitalized For Coronary Heart Disease," *The New England Journal of Medicine*, vol. 325, no. 4 (July 25, 1991), 224. See also Richard M. Steingart, M.D. and others, "Sex Differences in the Management of Coronary Artery Disease," *The New England Journal of Medicine*, vol. 325, no. 4 (July 25, 1991), 226-230.

unwarranted ignorance or limited intellectual capacity on the part of their patients and give a child's account of the situation. Or they clearly convey to the patient that they are very busy and do not have the time to spend on elaborate explanations. An even worse scenario of bad communication occurs when the doctor gives complete and accurate information, but in such technical language that the major part of the discourse sails right over the head of the bewildered patient. Both situations result in communication breakdowns and leave both parties frustrated and angry. A history of such unhappy medical encounters can make patients cynical and bitter, which can result in non-compliance at the very least, and sometimes, more seriously, in a total rejection of traditional medical practitioners for faith healers, witch doctors, and quacks. On the other hand, a history of unhappy patient encounters, particularly those in which the patient lied, or withheld information, can make the doctor equally suspicious and mistrustful. The ideal, of course, is Szasz's adult-to-adult relationship, but this ideal cannot come about unless doctors get off their pedestals and patients get off their knees. [6]

ii

Another dimension to the difficulties of coping with serious illness is money. Medical care in this country, while superb, is awesomely expensive. Doctor's fees are escalating daily, for many reasons. Most doctors have at least some new technology in their offices, such as computers, blood labs, and x-ray machines. This equipment is expensive, as is furniture, supplies, rent, and salaries for support staff. In addition, most doctors are passing on to the patient their escalating fees for liability insurance. These costs are legitimate, and account for much of the snowballing in doctors' bills. But much of it is also greed. Doctors enjoy a life-style far in excess of the average citizen, even those who are as highly educated. Whenever I am invited to lunch at our local country club, it is interesting to see the waiters greeting Doctor this and Doctor that, and they are not bestowing the title on Ph.D's. University Professors make a quarter of the average doctor's income, and seldom belong to country clubs. The traditional argument that doctors have to be compensated for their long years of training strikes me as a self-serving rationalization.

Hospital costs are also unbelievable. One of the reasons for hospital inflation, like that of doctors' bills, is expensive technology, but there is much duplication of equipment in hospitals and medical facilities down the street from each other. Hospitals also claim that they have to overcharge paying patients or patients with good insurance in order to offset those patients who do not pay. They call this cost-shifting, and such practices are the main reason that a pill you pay forty cents for at the drugstore costs five dollars in the hospital. Or you are charged ten dollars for a surgical dressing that is little more than a fifty-cent bandaid.

Another reason hospital bills are so astronomical is that many are now privately owned and operate for-profit. Insurance companies are increasingly restricting approved hospital stays, so hospitals must make up their profits by

[6]The phrase is not mine. I read it in a magazine in one of the countless doctors' waiting rooms I have been in over the past few years.

padding those bills of patients that must be hospitalized, or by charging appalling rates for outpatient procedures. For example, the bill for a cataract operation that I recently underwent as an outpatient at a local hospital was even more outrageous than usual. Much of the bill listed procedures and supplies that I did not understand, and I had no way of checking to make sure they were actually used or performed. Nor was I advised of the price list beforehand. But what really sent me into orbit was an appalling amount of money for seventeen, separately-listed, prescription drugs that they claim they gave me in the half-hour-long procedure. I insisted that the account be audited; they agreed, and appointed their own auditor to investigate my complaint. Once again, the proverbial wolf was sent in to guard the sheep pen. The auditor discovered one shot of Lidocaine for $16.50 that they didn't really use, and credited me for that amount.

The main difficulty with doctor and hospital costs is that the normal rules of supply and demand which usually keep down consumer costs do not operate in a medical setting. The consumer (patient) has no control over the selection of tests or drugs, and is not given a choice of alternatives based on costs. The doctor does all the ordering and demand-creating, oblivious for the most part, of the cost, supposedly for the good of the patient; but if the truth were known, many of the tests are to protect himself against lawsuits. Not only do doctors create the demand, they can charge as much as they want and as much as the traffic will bear. So can hospitals. The patient has little choice in the matter. I had no way of knowing if all the items listed in my cataract procedure bill were legitimate, or if the prices were reasonable.

Drugs are a slightly different matter. They have inflated some three hundred percent in the last few years, far, far more than the general rate of inflation. Drug companies justify their prices with the argument that they need to make large (huge?) profits in order to have the money to invest in costly research for new drugs. But as has recently been revealed, they spend far more on their advertising than they do on research. Again, the problem is monopoly. While they have the patent on the drug, they can charge whatever they will for it, and often do. AZT, the only drug that has as yet proven at all effective in retarding the advance of AIDS, was outrageously expensive when it first came out, until the government stepped in and insisted it be priced more reasonably. Once again, the situation smells strongly of greed.

Because of these wildly escalating costs, many people in this country simply cannot afford medical care. Indeed, our superb medical system is only available to those with money or with health insurance. And millions do not have either. Consequently, many simply do not go to the doctor and forego important treatment that could vastly improve the quality of their lives. Indeed, so severe is the crisis that we are facing the Orwellian possibility of rationed health care, where the more expensive procedures are reserved for the young who have a chance of returning to productive lives. In such a scenario, the elderly ill would be put on a maintenance program where they would be made comfortable until they died.

For those who do have the money, expensive medical treatment for a prolonged illness plunges them into bankruptcy. The resulting pressure breaks up families and involves the victim in a whirlpool of financial, psychological and, finally, physical breakdowns. Even those with health insurance suffer the same stresses. Premiums are escalating, benefits are being reduced or policies do not cover pre-existing conditions. And often, once the medical crisis is over, the insurance company cancels coverage for any future incidences of the same illness. I am among the lucky few who belong to a large group policy where the insurance company cannot drop me, nor restrict my claims for lupus. However, I still funnel a large portion of my monthly salary into insurance premiums, co-payments, deductibles and non-covered items. These expenses have severely qualified my life-style. The above situation is a national scandal, appalling for a nation that prides itself on being a world leader. Indeed, America must assume the moral and economic responsibility for its ill before it can preach its doctrines of democracy with any real credibility.

iii

A final dimension to the sufferings of the ill involves social attitudes. This work is not meant to be a sociological study of the effects of illness, but my personal confrontation with the situation has given me some startling insights into this area of human behavior that are worth sharing. In her deeply insightful book *Illness as Metaphor*, Susan Sontag traces nineteenth-century attitudes toward tuberculosis and twentieth-century attitudes toward cancer mainly by exploring how we use references to these two diseases as metaphors. The nineteenth century viewed tuberculosis as languishingly romantic, despite its devastating physical effects, and consequently the age coddled and supported its victims. The same is not true of cancer in the twentieth century. The term cancer, Sontag points out, is often used as a metaphor to describe a subtly encroaching evil, such as John Dean's reference to a "cancer" spreading on the presidency during the Watergate hearings. This highly pervasive and negative use of the metaphor has affected our attitudes toward cancer patients, and has qualified the way we treat them. Many people think of cancer as shameful, and even through we know it is not contagious, we avoid cancer victims the way we used to avoid those with leprosy.

Carrying Sontag's insights one step further, it is beginning to appear that, as we are slowly gaining on cancer, those with immune system diseases, particularly AIDS, are now the objects of fear and repugnance. Despite the massive attempt to educate people on the ways AIDS is transmitted, many still react to an AIDS sufferer in their midst with deep suspicion and sometimes even hysteria. So devastating is the current AIDS epidemic world-wide, it is now being referred to as the twentieth-century plague. And indeed, many people react with the same superstitions and irrational behaviors that our ancestors in the medieval world did. The high risk-groups, particularly homosexual men, have been identified almost exclusively with the disease, even though it is encroaching into the general population. Consequently, homosexuals are experiencing the same hysterical reactions and disgust from their fellow humans as did medieval sufferers of leprosy or the plague. We no longer ship them off to remote islands, or draw large red X's on their doors, but the scorn and horror and growing discrimination amounts to the same thing. And many consider their plight as God's just wrath on those who would indulge in deviant behavior, condemning them with a self-righteous scorn that is awesome.

Although AIDS is the current medical horror, all immune-system diseases are regarded with suspicion and fear. Many people have responded to the news that I have lupus with shock and usually blurt out their immediate reactions right in front of me. Most often the reaction is some form of query about it being contagious. And I know of many lupus sufferers who will not come to Lupus Association meetings because they are too deeply ashamed to come up front with their illness. Perhaps some of the deep-seated fear is in reaction to the elusiveness of immune-system problems. At least with cancer, you have a discernible tumor that can be felt and touched, and sometimes cut out. Not so with AIDS. The culprit is so small (a tiny virus) and so totally invasive, it is almost as if some evil being enters your body and slowly eats it away, cell by cell. In the case of autoimmune diseases, the idea of your own cells eating away at your body is just as repugnant. Another cause of the horror could also be the infinitesimally small size of the enemy and its ability to so totally take over one's body, almost like a demonic possession. The fear and horror of having something like that going on inside you is indescribable.

Another dimension to the social ramifications of being ill in twentieth-century America is the new wave of dealing with bodily functions and one's illness through mind control. The movement has many origins, but one of the most famous is the work of the Simonton's in Fort Worth, Texas. In their cancer clinic, they apply the theories of mind-body connection and the relationship between stress and illness to a formal course of treatment. Their approach is basically psychological and encourages the patient to think positively, to eliminate stress, to practice deep relaxation, to exercise and eat right, and mainly to begin visualizing, or imaging. This last technique has caught on around the country and involves visualizing some form of open-mouthed monster devouring the run-away cancer cells. They outline their therapy in their book *Getting Well Again*. This same approach can be found in countless other self-help books that have been glutting the book market in recent years, with perhaps the most sensible and thoroughly researched being Deepak Chopra's *Quantum Healing*. This approach has had enough success that clinics are springing up around the country teaching people relaxation and visualizing techniques as a way of dealing with any illness, not just cancer. Bernie Siegel's *Love, Medicine, and Miracles* is perhaps the most popular, and understandably so. His is a message to doctors as well as to patients about the curative effects of love and spiritual well-being. What makes his work superior to others of its type, to my mind, is his realization that death is a given. And that there comes a time when we have to accept the inevitable, either in our own lives, or that of loved ones. When this point is reached, Dr. Siegel strongly counsels either letting go oneself, or giving a loved one permission to let go. He rightly advocates putting the human factor back into the practice of medicine, and recapturing the compassionate and humane in our response to the seriously ill.

While there is much in this new movement that is unquestioningly good, it can also produce some unfortunate side effects. Because the patient is led to believe that he or she can control and even reverse the disease process through sheer effort of will, those patients who still become ill or further deteriorate are encouraged to believe that they are doing it to themselves. In other words, they are made to think they have brought on their own illness and are not getting better because they are not putting out the effort to mobilize the will, that they are what amounts to moral wimps. Even my own brother once remarked to me that I was still sick because I was not trying hard enough. It is difficult to put into words what that kind of attitude can do to a patient who is also struggling with the ravages of her disease, with health-care workers, and with financial disaster. While I certainly advocate putting up a fight against one's illness and often caution others about the dangers of the victim role, I am becoming more and more impatient with those who scorn the ill as somehow trying to cash in on the secondary gains of illness. While coping with serious illness certainly involves a commitment to aggressive participation in one's own health care, it also involves an ultimate acceptance of the inevitable, of that part of our illness that is, in the final analysis, beyond our control.

Being seriously ill, then, is a complex interdependent process that involves the sufferer in a comprehensive interplay of physical, psychological, economic, social and even spiritual conflicts. It is no wonder that the converging pressures plunge the ill into an abyss of despair and hopelessness. And it is ironic that the very system we have set up to help the ill has become part of the problem. Hopefully, as patients become more educated about medical matters and more responsible consumers, and doctors relinquish some of their power-hold over the practice of medicine in this country, some of this suffering associated with illness will be alleviated. But it is not possible to eliminate it entirely. It is best to remember that illness and death are a part of the human condition, and that the sick are deserving of our compassion and respectful awe, whatever their specific disease, as they endure their three-edged sword.

AFTERWORD

In the course of my sixteen-month odyssey, by far the worst time was my contact with the Mayo Clinic. Their failure to diagnose my illness was bad enough in itself, but labelling me as a possible psychiatric case was devastating. It took me many, many months to deal with the ramifications of their verdict, and I doubt that I will ever completely get over that terrible experience. I do not, however, maintain that the Mayo Clinic is an incompetent institution. On the contrary, its reputation as one of the finest medical centers in our country is justly deserved. It attracts the brightest and best of medical graduates, and can boast of top-flight specialists in every field. In addition, the Mayo Clinic's record of significant research is sterling. Further, the sheer volume of patients that go through the clinic (twelve hundred on one day I was there, so a lab technician told me), guarantees that the Mayo Clinic doctors will be exposed to and learn from just about every ill that can afflict humankind. Because these doctors have had such a broad range of experience, their track record on accurate diagnosis is remarkably fine. Finally, the Mayo Clinic has some of the best and latest in diagnostic equipment modern science has developed. Indeed, because of its remarkable successes and contributions to the field of medicine, the Mayo Clinic has justly become a world-wide beacon of hope, a court of last appeal, the ultimate source of stunning medical expertise.

There is a serious danger, however, that the absolute faith most people have in the Mayo Clinic will result in the myth of omnipotence and omniscience. While such legendary fame may be flattering to the institution or to individual doctors who work there, it also gives them a terrible power over our lives, and an awesome responsibility. And when that power and responsibility are abused, the result is a suffocating arrogance that is destructive to everyone concerned. It is for this reason that I did not change the name or attempt in any way to conceal the identity of this institution. The appalling consequences I suffered from their treatment of me would not have been so severe, had it been just any clinic. I went to Rochester, as do so many people, utterly convinced that my problems would be resolved, that "they" would find out what was wrong with me, that I would be cured, and that I could get on with my life. After all, it was *the* Mayo Clinic. In part then, I must also share the blame for the shattering results. I learned many things from this experience, but perhaps the most important lesson I have come away with is my new-found awareness that Medicine does not have all the answers, nor can it do all things. In the final analysis, it is the individual patient who must take charge of his or her own life, to take responsibility for the outcome, and not to put the burden elsewhere.

A SELECT BIBLIOGRAPHY

Aladjem, H. and Peter H. Shur, M.D. *In Search of the Sun: A Woman's Courageous Victory Over Lupus*. New York: Charles Scribner's Sons, 1988.

----------. *Understanding Lupus: What It Is, How To Treat It, How To Cope With It*. New York: Charles Scribner's Sons, 1985.

Albrecht, Gary L. and Paul C. Higgins, eds. *Health, Illness and Medicine: A Reader in Medical Sociology*. Chicago: Rand McNally College Publishing Company, 1979.

The American Medical Association Family Medical Guide. Editor-in chief Jeffrey R.M. Kunz, M.D. New York: Random House, 1982.

Anderson, Timothy and David Helm. "The Physician-Patient Encounter." In *Patients, Physicians and Illness: A Sourcebook in Behavioral Science and Health*, 3rd. ed., edited by E. Gartly Jaco, 259-271. New York: The Free Press, 1979.

Ayanian, John Z., M.D. and Arnold M. Epstein, M.D. "Differences in the Use of Procedures Between Women and Men Hospitalized for Coronary Heart Disease." *The New England Journal of Medicine* 325 no.4(July 25, 1991): 221-225.

Apple, Dorrian. "How Laymen Define Illness." *Journal of Health and Social Behavior* 1(1961): 219-225.

Argyle, Michael. *Social Skills and Health*. New York: Methuen, 1981.

Beatty, J. and H. Legewie, eds. *Biofeedback and Behavior*. New York: Plenum, 1977.

Bennet, Glin. *Patients and Their Doctors: The Journey Through Medical Care*. London: Bailliere Tindall, 1979.

Benson, H. *The Relaxation Response*. New York: William Morrow and Company, 1975.

Blackie, Margery Grace. *The Patient, Not the Cure*. London: Macdonald and Jane's, 1976.

Bloom, S.W. *The Doctor and His Patient: A Sociological Interpretation*. New York: Russell Sage Foundation, 1963.

Bronson, L. "Former Patient at Angews 'Tells It Like It Was.'" *Palo Alto Times*, June 21, 1972: 27.

Brown, B.D. *I Choose to Live*! Nashville, TN: Winston-Derek Publishers, 1990.

Brown, Esther. *Patients As People*. New York: Russell Sage Foundation, 1964.
Buchanan, James H. *Patient Encounters: The Experience of Disease*. Virginia: University of Virginia Press, 1989.
Cartwright, Ann. *Patients and Their Doctors*. New York: Atherton Press, 1967.
Chopra, Deepak. *Quantum Healing: Exploring the Frontiers of Body, Mind, Medicine*. New York: Bantam Books, 1990
Cleveland, Martha. *The Twelve Step Response To Chronic Illness and Disability: Recovering Joy in Life*. Maryland: Hazelden, 1988.
Cousins, Norman. *Anatomy of An Illness*. New York: W.W. Norton, 1979.
---------------. *The Healing Heart: Antidotes to Panic and Helplessness*. New York: W.W. Norton, 1983.
Cook, I.S. *The Victim is Always the Same*. New York: Harper and Row, 1973.
Ehrenreich, John. *The Cultural Crisis of Modern Medicine*. New York: Monthly Review Press, 1978.
Folta, Jeannette R. and Edith S. Deck. *A Sociological Framework for Patient Care*. New York: John Wiley and Sons, 1966.
Frances, V., B.M. Korsch, and M.T. Moris. "Gaps in Doctor-Patient Communication: Patients' Response to Medical Advice." *New England Journal of Medicine* 280 (March 16, 1969): 535-540.
Freeman, B. et al. "Gaps in Doctor-Patient Communication: Doctor-Patient Interaction Analyses." *Pediatric Research*, July 5, 1971: 298-311.
Friedman, Howard and Robin Di Matteo. *Interpersonal Issues in Health Care*. New York: Harper and Row, 1968.
Fromm, E. *The Revolution of Hope: Toward a More Humanized Technology*. New York: Harper and Row, 1968.
Gallagher, Eugene F. "Lines of Reconstruction and Extension in the Parsonian Sociology of Illness." In *Patients, Physicians and Illness: A Sourcebook in Behavioral Science and Health*, 3rd. ed. Edited by E. Gartly Jaco, 202-217. New York: The Free Press, 1979.
Geiger, Jack. H., M.D. "The Causes of Dehumanization in Health Care and Prospects for Humanization." In *Humanizing Health Care*. Edited by Jan Howard and Anselm Strauss, 11-36. New York: John Wiley and Sons, 1978.
Gerhardt, Uta. *Ideas about Illness: An Intellectual and Political History of Medical Sociology*. New York: New York University Press, 1989.
Gray, Henry, F.R.S., *Atanomy: Descriptive and Surgical*, edited by T. Pickering Pick and Robert Howden. New York: Bounty Books, 1977
Gunther, John. *Death Be Not Proud*. New York: Pyramid, 1962.
Halberstam, Michael and Stephan Lesher. *A Coronary Event*. Philadelphia: J.B. Lippincott, 1976.
Hamo, A. "The Incredible Ordeal of Chad Calland, M.D." *Redbook* 137 (September, 1971).
Hollender, Marc H. *The Psychology of Medical Practice*. Philadelphia: W.B Saunders Co., 1958.
Howard, Jan and Anselm Strauss, eds. *Humanizing Health Care*. New York: John Wiley and Sons, 1975.
Jaco, E. Gartly, ed. *Patients, Physicians, and Illness: A Sourcebook in Behavioral Science and Health*. 3rd ed. New York: The Free Press, 1979.
Kesey, Ken. *One Flew Over the Cuckoo's Nest*. New York: Signet, 1962.

Korsch, B.M. and V.F. Nigrette. "Doctor-Patient Communication." *Scientific American*, 22 (August, 1972): 66-74.
Knutson, Andie L. *The Individual, Society and Health Behavior*. New York: Russell Sage Foundation, 1965.
Krause, Elliott A. *Power and Illness: The Political Sociology of Health and Medical Care*. New York: Elsevier, 1977.
Kubler-Ross, Elizabeth. *On Death and Dying*. New York: The Macmillan Co., 1969.
Kushner, Irving, M.D., Ann Forer and Ann B. McGuire, eds. *Understanding Arthritis*. Arthritis Foundation. New York: Charles Scribner's Sons, 1984.
Fox, Marion Laffey. *A Patient Guide to Medical Testing*. Charles Press Publishers, 1979.
Leigh, Hoyle and Morton F. Reiser. *The Patient: Biological, Psychological and Social Dimensions of Medical Practice*. 2nd. ed. New York: Plenum Publishers, 1985.
Lewis, K. S. *Successful Living With Chronic Illness*. Wayne, NJ: Avery Publishing Group, 1985.
Lipp, Martin R., M.D. *The Bitter Pill: Doctors, Patients, and Failed Expectations*. New York: Harper and Row, 1980.
Lupkin, Mack. "On Lying to Patients." *Newsweek* (June 4, 1979): 13.
Lorber, Judith. "Good Patients and Problem Patients: Conformity and Deviance in a General Hospital." In *Patients, Physicians and Illness: A Sourcebook in Behavioral Science and Health*. 3rd ed. Edited by E. Gartly Jaco, 202-217. New York: The Free Press, 1979.
Mechanic, David and M. Zborowski. *People in Pain*. San Francisco: Jossey-Bass, 1969.
Mechanic, David. *Medical Sociology*. 2nd. ed. New York: The Free Press, 1978.
---------------. "Social Psychological Factors Affecting the Presentation of Bodily Complaints." *The New England Journal of Medicine* 286 (May, 1972): 1132-1139.
Nolen, William. *A Surgeon Under the Knife*. New York: Coward McCann and Geoghegan, Inc., 1976.
Nouwen, Henri. *The Wounded Healer: Ministry in Contemporary Society*. New York: Doubleday, 1979.
O'Connor, Flannery. *A Habit of Being: Letters of Flannery O'Connor*. Edited by Sally Fitzgerald. New York: Farrar, Straus and Giroux, 1978.
Park, Clara. *You Are Not Alone*. Boston: Atlantic-Little, Brown, 1976.
Parker, A.W. "The Consumer as Policy-Maker: Issues of Training." *American Journal of Public Health* 60 (November, 1970): 2139-2153.
Parsons, Talcott. "Illness and the Role of the Physician." *Journal of Orthopsychiatry* 21 (July, 1951): 452-460.
---------------. "Definitions of Health and Illness in the Light of American Values and Social Structure." *Patients, Physicians, and Illness: A Sourcebook in Behavioral Science and Health*. 3rd ed. Edited by E. Gartly Jaco, 120-144. New York: The Free Press, 1979.
Patterson, Richard B. *In Search of the Wounded Healer: A Helping Professional's Guide to Inner Resources*. New Jersey: Dimension Books, 1990.

Pelletier, K. R. *Mind as Healer, Mind as Slayer*. New York: Delta, 1977.

Permut, J.B. *Embracing the Wolf*. Georgia: Cherokee Publishing Company, 1989.

Phillips, Robert H. *Coping With Lupus: A Guide to Living with Lupus for You and Your Family*. New Jersey: Avery Publishing Group, 1984.

Pinner, Max and Benjamin Millers, eds. *When Doctors are Patients*. New York: W.W. Norton, 1952.

Pitzele, Sefra Kobrin. *We Are Not Alone: Learning to Live With Chronic Illness*. New York: Workman Publishing, 1985.

Radziunas, E. *Lupus: My Search for a Diagnosis*. Claremont, CA: Hunter House Inc., Publishers, 1989.

Ramsey, Paul. *The Patient as Person: Explorations in Medical Ethics*. New Haven: Yale University Press, 1969.

Rogers, Malcolm P. "Clinical Aspects." In "*The Clinical Management of Systemic Lupus Erythematosus*. Edited by Peter H. Shur M.D. Florida: Grune & Stratton, 1983.

Rosenbaum, Edward E. *A Taste of My Own Medicine: When the Doctor is the Patient* New York: Random House, 1988.

Ryan, William. *Blaming the Victim*. New York: Pantheon Books, 1971.

Schur, Peter H. M.D. ed., *The Clinical Management of Systemic Lupus Erythematosus*. Florida: Grune & Stratton, 1983.

Siegel, Bernie S. *Love, Medicine and Miracles: Lessons Learned About Self-Healing From a Surgeon's Experience With Exceptional Patients*. New York: Harper and Row, 1986.

Siegler, Miriam. *Patienthood: The Art of Being a Responsible Patient*. New York: Macmillan, 1979.

Seligman, M.E.P. *Helplessness: On Depression, Development, and Death*. San Francisco: W.H. Freeman and Co., 1975.

Selye, Hans. *The Stress of Life*. New York: McGraw-Hill, 1956.

Simonton, O. Carl, M.D., Stephanie Matthews-Simonton and James L. Creighton. *Getting Well Again: A Step by Step Guide to Overcoming Cancer for Patients and Their Families*. New York: Bantam Books, 1980.

Skipper, J.K. Jr., and R.C. Leonard, eds. *Social Interaction and Patient Care*. Philadelphia: Lippincott, 1965.

Slaby, Andrew Edmund, M.D., and Arvin Sigmund Glicksman, M.D. *Adapting to Life Threatening Illness*. New York: Praeger Publishers, 1985.

Smith, D.E. and J. Luce. *Love Needs Care*. Boston: Little Brown, 1971.

Solzhenitsyn, A.I. *Cancer Ward*. New York: Harper and Row, 1969.

Steingart, Richard M. et al. "Sex Differences in the Management of Coronary Artery Disease." *The New England Journal of Medicine* 325, no. 4 (July 25, 1991): 226-230.

Szasz, Thomas S. "Malingering: Diagnosis or Social Condemnation." *AMA Archaeology, Neurology and Psychiatry* 76 (1956) 432ff.

-----------. *The Myth of Mental Illness*. New York: Harper and Row, 1961.

-----------. "Illness and Indignity." *Journal of the American Medical Association* 227 (February 4, 1974): 543-545.

Tagliacozzo, Daisy L. and Hans O. Mauksch. "The Patient's View of the Patient's Role." *Patients, Physicians and Illness: A Sourcebook in Behavioral Science and Health*. 3rd ed. Edited by E. Gartly Jaco, 184-201. New York: The Free Press, 1979.

Taylor, Shelly E. "Hospital Patient Behavior: Reactance, Helplessness, or Control?" *Interpersonal Issues in Health Care*. Edited by Howard S. Friedman and M. Robin DiMatteo, 209-232. New York: Academic Press, 1982.

Virshum, Bernard. *How to Cope With Your Doctor*. San Bernardino, California: Borgo Press, 1985.

INDEX